No germs allowed!

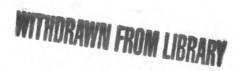

No germs allowed!

How to avoid infectious diseases at home and on the road

Revised and expanded edition

Winkler G. Weinberg, MD

RUTGERS UNIVERSITY PRESS
New Brunswick, New Jersey

Library of Congress Cataloging-in-Publication Data

Weinberg, Winkler G., 1952–
    No germs allowed! : how to avoid infectious diseases at home and
on the road / by Winkler G. Weinberg.—Rev. & expanded ed.
      p. cm.
    Includes bibliographical references and index.
    ISBN 0-8135-3532-8 (pbk. : alk. paper)
    1. Travel—Health aspects. 2. Communicable diseases—Prevention.
3. Infection. I. Title.
    RA783.5.W44 2004
    616.9'045—dc22
                                          2004050955
                                                CIP

British Cataloging-in-Publication information available

To my talented, dedicated, and loving wife, Lynn

Contents

Appendixes

Tables and figures

Tables

Figures

Acknowledgments

First and foremost I would like to thank the editor of my first edition, Dr. Karen Reeds, and the editor of the present edition, Dr. Audra Wolfe. Each is dedicated to science, accuracy, and service to others. Without their support and literary expertise, these books could not have been completed. Similarly, without the help of copyeditor Kate Fuller, this manuscript would be immeasurably less readable and understandable. I also greatly appreciate the guidance and coordination of Marilyn Campbell, prepress director.

Lynn Weinberg and Annette Joseph prepared several of the illustrations and assisted with others. Their talent and efforts are greatly appreciated. I also thank Eve Weinberg, who helped with the artwork, and Gabriel Weinberg, whose computer expertise and advice were indispensable.

The comments of a number of critical readers were invaluable. These included: Evelyn Sacks; Dr. Cynthia Gilbert; Dr. Fred Gordon; Dr. Jane Geltner; Dr. Sidney Weinberg; Emily Mendel; Janice Reece; Dr. Frank Joseph; Dr. Lee Jacobs; Diane Weyer, CFNP; Gayle Arberg, CANP; and Dr. Edward C. Oldfield III.

Acknowledgments

No germs allowed!

Introduction: At risk

It's the time of your life. It's the ultimate getaway. Despite months of stress, both on and off the job, you're finally on your way! This time it's your turn—the chance you've waited for. Time to go as far away as possible and do things you've never done before. Off to the backcountry and beyond.

The adventure tour is incredible. Your guide's terrific. He won't allow you to miss a thing. The group sleeps in on the fifth morning, but stays late in the bush to make up for it. You ford the local river to reach a great spot for viewing wildlife. Unfortunately, the mosquitoes are more active than the animals you've come to see. Still, the river crossing is pleasant in bare feet, and the scene of the villagers washing their clothes just upstream will make a great photo. Tramping on, you forget the mosquitoes because the flies, ticks, and dust are even more bothersome! Nevertheless, the sunset was the experience of a lifetime.

Two more days in, though, and you're wallowing in doubt, as well as mud. This Alaska, Galapagos, jungle, "see the whale," and "add one to your life list" circuit is really not for you. You've had your fill of dung, bugs, and potholes. You long for a city. The tour includes another three days in the bush, but you decide to spend them in town and perhaps rub elbows with the locals. It's a hot two and a half hours on a bus filled with crying babies and coughing adults, and there are long waits at cattle crossings, but, yes, you do get a chance to immerse yourself in the real world.

Who wants to be alone at night in a strange city? You know you should be careful, but you desperately want to get out.

You go to the hotel lobby where you soon find another solo traveler who is glad to join you for dinner.

Happily, your new acquaintance frequents this city on business and takes you on a brief tour. Afterward, you dine at a romantic continental restaurant, with ceviche and steak tartare for appetizers, salad niçoise, and delicious pork tenderloin. The champagne is local but excellent. The only letdown comes with your request for iced tea—disappointed, you accede to instant. But the cappuccino that accompanies dessert is perfect.

The next night is equally charming. You feel there is a bond developing that you would like to solidify. You share an intimate, passionate night at the Intercontinental Hotel and ride together to the airport the next morning. You exchange parting thoughts about the future while your jets take on fuel, food, and water. As you board, you feel positively energized, as though you're taking with you living portions of the backcountry, the plains, and your lover. (Indeed, you are!)

As we step back from this fantasy vacation, we wave good-bye and wish "best of luck" to our fictional traveler—who has been exposed to more than thirty-five infectious diseases in the course of this adventure. Later I'll return to our story to revisit the specific points where the traveler was at risk of acquiring infection. For now, let's consider the sobering and somewhat frightening fact that more than twenty-five of the diseases have nothing to do with foreign travel and could have been picked up just as easily in southern California, Ohio, Florida, Vancouver, or just about anywhere in North America.

Infection is everywhere. We live in continual contact with microorganisms in our environment and carry billions of bacteria and viruses within us always. Most of us are usually protected from becoming ill in this environment by an intact immune system. However, if we allow ourselves to contact a particularly virulent microorganism that is adept at evading our defenses, or if our immune system becomes impaired, an infectious disease can develop. In most cases, the infection is preventable.

When I see patients with such avoidable illness, I feel the impulse to scream, "How idiotic and careless you were! This infection was totally unnecessary!" Fortunately, a decade of postgraduate training and another two decades of medical practice have given me a somewhat more refined bedside manner. Besides, the scolding would be misplaced. A more appropriate outburst would be, "Why didn't anybody tell you?" The answer would be that the information needed to prevent infection in the first place is generally not readily available.

People tend to become educated about diseases after they've already contracted them and are ill. That's the way our current health care system works—contacts with professionals are interventional, not preventive. Preventive care visits often are not covered by insurance plans. Also, that's the way of human nature. Most of us do not usually seek medical advice when we are feeling well. (Health maintenance organizations may be slowly turning this around, encouraging and covering preventive care.) Despite these obstacles, in the high-stakes world of infectious disease, prevention is much simpler, much less painful, much less costly, and much safer than treatment.

It is in this spirit that I have written this book, attempting to make this important information about preventing disease readable, if not intriguing. Risk-averse readers will benefit most by reading the book through. Those with a particular interest— for example, the spouse of someone with hepatitis or someone whose tuberculosis skin test has converted to positive—will find that each chapter can stand alone.

This book is meant to be practical. One way I have tried to keep it practical is by emphasizing those infections that should be of most concern to Americans. We often find diseases that are sensational, frightening, or new featured in the media. Plague, hantavirus, and Ebola virus are such infections. Although they are serious and important ailments, the average American, even the adventuresome traveler, is at nearly no risk from such dangers. For example, no tourists (and probably very few Indian nationals) developed plague after the 1994 outbreak in Surat, India. Fewer than 500 people have developed hantavirus pulmonary syndrome to date. And no cases of Ebola hemorrhagic fever occurred outside the area around Kikwit, Zaire, in 1995. (Ebola is actually quite hard to catch. Only 17 percent of household contacts came down with the disease, and these persons had had close contacts with infected family members.) So, although I will discuss the prevention of some of these rare but dramatic infections, my main focus is infections for which Americans are at some substantial risk.

Let's return to our traveler, who so far is lucky. However, it would be a miracle if this asymptomatic state persisted for too long. The notion of taking bits of life home is likely to be as literal as it is romantic. Our traveler's tropical itinerary involved risk for many infections—most of them not exclusively tropical. For example, wading through a stream in many African, Latin American, or Asian countries will put you at serious risk of getting a parasitic disease called schistosomiasis. Several Harvard students acquired schistosomiasis in Egypt in the late 1980s; one became paraplegic as a result. However, just as you can easily pick up malaria or typhus from mosquito or flea bites while traveling in India, closer to home mosquito and tick bites might give you eastern equine encephalitis while you're watching a Florida sunset, Rocky Mountain spotted fever when you're camping in North Carolina, Lyme disease while you're mowing the lawn in Connecticut, or West Nile virus.

An infection's incubation period is the time it takes after a microorganism enters a person's body until the victim feels ill. Incubation periods can be quite short or quite long. When the coleslaw for the Saturday church picnic is carefully laid out two hours early by a parishioner, the congregation may be vomiting from staphylococcal food poisoning before the softball game's over. (Luckily, they'll all recover in time for Sunday morning services.) However, a bite to the foot by a rabid animal—as far removed from the central nervous system as you can get—could have an incubation period of years—as many as nineteen and a half years, one case report suggests.

Although our traveler felt quite well boarding the flight home, he or she might have been incubating several infections at that time. The astute reader shuddered during the terrifying scene in our story when the protagonist innocently spends two and a half hours in an enclosed space (on a bus) with coughing local inhabitants. Although this puts the traveler at risk for any number of airborne diseases, tuberculosis (TB) is the greatest worry. (Note that a bus ride in Los Angeles could present the same hazard.) TB's incubation period can also be years long (see chapter 9), but the disease might already be brewing on the flight home. Likewise, the dust inhaled on the safari might have contained the spores of *Histoplasma capsulatum.* Histoplasmosis is a fungal pneumonia with an incubation period of two weeks; you could also contract it on a dusty excursion in Missouri. A similar fungal infection, coccidioidomycosis, is common in Arizona and California (see chapter 8). The instant iced tea served to our traveler at dinner could have presented a double whammy (see chapter 7). If mixed with local tap water, the garden varieties of traveler's diarrhea would have been likely. These have a short incubation period. But even if the tea had been made with boiled or bottled water, the ice could have been laced with cysts of an ameba or of *Giardia.* The incubation periods of these infections are weeks long, and would not be likely to send the traveler running to the bathroom until he or she was back home, reviewing the photos.

I won't dwell on all the rare diseases our story brings to

mind, but they are generally unpleasant. They include mosquito-borne encephalitis as well as onchocerciasis, or "river blindness," transmitted by the bites of black flies along riverbanks. Also, from the gourmet dinner our traveler could have picked up parasites from raw fish in the ceviche, toxoplasmosis from the steak tartare, amebic cysts on the lettuce in the salad niçoise, and trichinosis in the rare pork tenderloin (see chapter 6).

Perhaps traveler's diarrhea, or any of the milder infections with a short incubation period, might have been a blessing in disguise. If the second date had been canceled because of illness, the risk of contracting herpes, syphilis, gonorrhea, chlamydia, chancroid, and quite a number of other sexually transmitted diseases (STDs) might have been avoided (see chapter 10). Not to mention HIV, the cause of AIDS (chapter 12).

To prevent and avoid infection, you must first understand something of the infecting organism and its life cycle. This book is designed to give you that basic information. To accomplish that, a few basic definitions are essential. I have already mentioned that an infectious disease is an illness caused by a microorganism, that is, a virus, bacterium, protozoan, or parasite. Yet not all infectious diseases are "catching," meaning contagious or communicable; for example, urinary tract infections. Urinary tract infections occur when your own normal bowel bacteria ascend into the bladder where they ought not to be. Feces are more bacterial than undigested food and contain ten billion to a hundred billion bacteria per ounce. When confined to their usual home, these bowel florae cause no illness, but assist in the normal function of the large intestine.

So, can you be infected but not have a contagious or infectious disease? Have an infectious disease and not be contagious? Be contagious but not infected? We'd better digress.

For you to be infected, an organism need only take up residence in your body. It need not be causing an illness or disease. It need not be transmissible to another person. For example, if you are over thirty, there is a 90 percent chance you are infected with the herpes simplex virus. Chances are, it is residing comfortably in a latent state in some of the nerve cells next to your spinal cord. It is not hurting you and you can't give it to anyone. In this case you would be infected but not have a disease, and you would not be contagious.

Now plan a family trip to the beach. If you don't put on a lip balm with sunscreen, the sunshine signals the herpes virus to start growing again (termed reactivation), and before you know it you have a fever blister. That cluster of tiny blisters just outside the red of your lip impairs your normal state. Congratulations. You now have an infectious disease. It is not serious and you didn't have to do anything risky or stupid to get it, but it is an illness nonetheless.

Are you now contagious? Yes. While the virus was tucked away in the nerve cell it had no way to contact another human being. Now that it has grown down the nerve and out to the surface of the skin it has plenty of opportunity. You are now contagious and the disease you have is communicable; you can pass the virus to another individual. Young children around you are very likely to pick up herpes simplex virus and very unlikely to even know they have done so. However, if your teenager and/or spouse are still uninfected and get a kiss from you, you may end up feeding them soup and ice cream in bed for a week. After returning home from the beach, they may need that long to recover from primary herpetic gingivostomatitis, a sometimes severe and extensive mouth infection characterized by ulcers. At different times and under different conditions, the same virus can cause widely different syndromes. I will try to point out this sort of nuance in each chapter.

I've personally cared for patients with each infection mentioned in this book. These diseases are real. I don't want you to get them. That's why I wrote this book. However, I don't want to spoil your fun either! After you've read this book, it is my hope and expectation that you will be able to travel nearly wherever you want, eat nearly anything you want, and even have an active sex life, but still not end up as one of my future case histories. Remember: most infections are avoidable.

One

The infections of daily living

1   *The common cold*

Among infections, upper respiratory tact infections (URIs) are the most common, although they're rarely serious. Whenever surveys are taken of households in the United States, URIs are by far the most frequent medical problem reported. The average preschool child has six to ten URIs each year and adults have two to four of them each year. Women, probably because of their exposure to young children, get more URIs than men. Millions of visits are made to doctors, millions of days are lost from work, and billions of dollars are spent on remedies for URIs every year.

A URI, though, is not one particular disease. Many—actually, hundreds—of different kinds of germs, mostly viruses, can infect your nose, throat, and other parts of your upper airways. But the most frequent offender is a tiny virus called the rhinovirus. (*Rhino* is Greek for nose.) This tiny virus causes the most typical form of what we call the common cold.

As its name implies, a typical rhinovirus infection will primarily torment you in your nose. This virus grows best in the somewhat cooler temperatures found there; it grows poorly at core body temperature (at 98.6°F or 37°C), so it does not invade deeper structures. An infected nose runs a clear or mucoid fluid and feels not only congested but blocked. The tip of the nose may turn red as well. A sore or scratchy throat is common, cough and hoarseness are not infrequent, but actual fever (over 100°F) is unusual. You can expect to improve in three or four days and get over a rhinovirus infection mostly in about a week, with some exceptions. (If you smoke, then the illness, especially the cough, may be prolonged.) On the tail end of a rhinovirus infection you become likely to develop sinusitis or an ear infection. The sinuses and ears must drain freely into the nose and throat in order to remain uninfected, and the swelling that occurs with a cold can block those passageways.

The set of symptoms that I've described for you characterizes the common cold, and most often, the common cold is a rhinovirus infection. However, many of the other viruses and some of the bacteria that cause URIs can mimic this picture. More often, they're less characteristic; the variations in symptoms of URI are innumerable. Much of what we know, though, about how one gets a URI relates particularly to rhinovirus and is thanks to the studies of Dr. Jack Gwaltney, an experimental virologist at the University of Virginia. Much of what I'm going to say about transmission comes from his work.

Rhinovirus is seasonal. Most years, especially on the East Coast, many people tend to catch cold in the fall, usually in September. Another but less prominent wave of colds often occurs in March, April, or May. These may be the common cold seasons because they are also the wet seasons, and rhinoviruses survive better outside our bodies when the humidity is high. Also, we spend more time indoors then: children go back to school in September, and as we congregate, we facilitate the spread of the virus. Contrary to popular belief, the increase of colds in the fall is probably not directly related to the weather. Volunteers exposed to cold temperatures show no more susceptibility to rhinovirus infection than their comfortable counterparts do. People of all ages get colds, but children and young adults get the most.

You can pick up a cold from anyone with whom you share close quarters. You are much more likely to catch a cold at home or at school than you are at work, at the mall, or on the train. How does rhinovirus get from one person to another? First, it gets on your hands. Then, you rub it into your eyes and nose. In the course of our daily activities, we are constantly touching our eyes and our nose, often unknowingly: this is normal behavior (see figure 1.1). But if rhinovirus is present on our hands, it can be the start of a cold. How does the rhinovirus get to your hands in the first place? You can pick it up when you touch another person (for example, shake hands or care for a child) or touch something in your immediate environment (the doorknob, for example, or the telephone). Rhinovirus can survive for over twenty-four hours on objects and surfaces.

Hand-to-nose transfer of germs may be the most common way to get colds, but you can also catch a cold through the air. A geyser of large and small particles will erupt from an uncovered sneeze or cough (see figure 1.2). These particles can directly infect you by landing in your eye or in your nose, or they can contaminate the surfaces you will soon touch.

Let me make some suggestions—some readily apparent—about how not to catch rhinovirus colds. Naturally, you should encourage people with colds to cover their mouth and nose

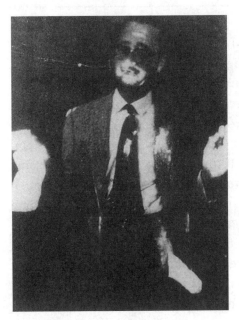

FIGURE 1.1 *Spreading a cold by touching*
A fluorescent dye was placed in this man's nose six hours earlier. The areas that are now glowing under fluorescent light show all the places he touched on his person: his hands, face, handkerchief, and clothes. If he had a cold, the rhinovirus would be on all these places, ready to be spread to other people and surfaces. Likewise, if he had picked up rhinovirus on his hands, he would have spread it to his own nose.

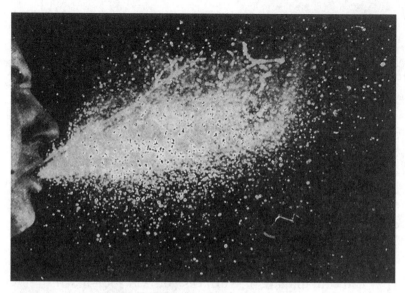

FIGURE 1.2 *Spreading a cold by sneezing*
Small droplets, large droplets, and strings of mucus are ejected from the mouth during a sneeze. This person has a cold and is contaminating his environment with rhinovirus.
Source: M. W. Jennison, *Aerobiology,* vol. 17 (Washington, D.C.: 1942): 106. American Association for the Advancement of Science; reprinted by permission.

well when they cough and sneeze. They should be using disposable tissues. Depending on how vigilant you want to be, it may be helpful to use a germicide to clean household surfaces that you suspect have become contaminated. Frequent hand washing or use of a hand sanitizer is also a good idea, whenever hands may have been contaminated.

It would be wonderful if these were a safe and inexpensive substance you could take to prevent colds. Unfortunately, such a brew has not been concocted. But naturally, when two-time Nobel Prize winner Linus Pauling published *Vitamin C and the Common Cold* in 1970, people were ready to believe. At that time, headlines were made, and vitamin C (ascorbic acid) became so popular that pharmacies were unable to maintain adequate supplies. However, no experimental data were available, only theories. Now, decades and fourteen studies later, it had been clearly shown that vitamin C (ascorbic acid) does not prevent a cold. It is also of little use, if any, in treating a cold. However, just as retractions never have the impact of erroneous headlines, I know that some readers will remain unshaken in their conviction that they feel better and are less ill with respiratory illnesses when they drink orange juice or take vitamin C. They should be careful not to overdo it. Vitamin C in megadoses (more than two grams per day) can lead to kidney stones. Everything from A to Z has been tried for the common cold, but there is no good evidence that any of them, from aspirin to echinacea to zinc, will be of any benefit.

2 ___ *Strep throat and other strep infections*

*I*t's a funny thing how two people, owing to their different aims and past experiences, can look at the very same situation and see it in two very different ways. This happens when you have a sore throat and visit a doctor. You might be thinking that you have a minor medical nuisance and want only to get rid of it with the least investment of time and expense. You probably suspect that taking antibiotic pills for a few days will accomplish that. The doctor wants the same positive and expedient outcome for you, but at the same time is asking some (often unspoken) further questions: Since most cases of inflamed throat (pharyngitis) are caused by viruses, and since antibiotics won't affect viruses, would treating you just put you at risk for side effects? If it is a viral infection, could it be infectious mononucleosis, which improves much more slowly than other viral infections? If it does turn out to be a strep throat—that is, an infection caused by bacteria—could you develop any of its complications: an abcess behind the throat or tonsil, invasion of the bloodstream, or the diseases of heart and kidney (rheumatic fever and glomerulonephritis) that sometimes follow strep infections? But some questions should be asked by both patient and doctor: Where did this illness come from? How can we be sure not to spread it around? How best to avoid a recurrence?

The tonsils are really the infection-fighting glands of your throat, so tonsillitis and pharyngitis are really one and the same. If the redness, swelling, tenderness, and sometimes pus occur primarily in the back of the throat we tend to call the illness pharyngitis. And if the symptoms are off to the side and over the tonsil(s), it may be called tonsillitis. Wherever the sore throat is centered, if a bacterium is the cause, the most common culprit is *Streptococcus pyogenes*, alias group A streptococci. This particular germ is the cause not only of strep throat but of many other human maladies as well, ranging from common impetigo (see chapter 4) to what the press termed "flesh-eating bacteria" (which we will discuss a little later).

Although streptococcal throat infections are most common in school-aged children, they can happen at any age. Kids get one, on average, every three to five years, but streptococci can also infect the kids' parents. Adults living in crowded quarters, like dorms, camps, and barracks, are particularly vulnerable. Strep infections have even spread through nursing homes.

If you get strep throat, your symptoms may be only a scratchy throat and temporary malaise, but typically they'll be worse. Most commonly, starting one to four days after you've been exposed to group A strep bacteria, the sore throat will start abruptly, often accompanied by fever and headache. The glands just below the angle of your jaw may become tender and swollen and you may see white or gray pus on your tonsils or throat.

Streptococcal pharyngitis spreads by direct contact or through the air. It is often carried by hands that have been near an infected person's mouth. It also can travel in the large droplets produced by a person who coughs. It often spreads through a household, usually within the first fourteen days after someone brings it home.

Obviously, in order to avoid catching strep throat, you need to avoid contact with anyone who has an untreated sore throat, and you don't want them to cough on you. Sometimes, though, this is a tall order. It's the kids who usually bring it home, so families with school-aged children are going to have a hard time staying strep-free. However, you are not totally defenseless against *Streptococcus pyogenes.* Your best weapon is penicillin. This is one germ that has not yet learned to foil penicillin. (If you're allergic, there are also good alternatives.) Within twenty-four hours of starting treatment, you or your family member will no longer be contagious, so get strep throat treated promptly.

There are two other reasons why you must seek prompt and proper treatment for streptococcal pharyngitis. With treatment, you will not only prevent its spreading to other people, but you will also prevent its spreading within you. Without treatment, the strep germs can form an abscess behind your throat or can lead to infections of your ears, sinuses, or lymph glands, and can even cause pneumonia. Then, there are later complications of group A streptococcal infection that can be quite serious. These occur because proteins on the surface of some of the strep bacteria are quite similar to proteins on the surface of our heart valves and kidney cells. So, when your immune system dutifully makes antibodies to fight off your strep infection, there's a small chance the antibodies will mistake your heart or your kidneys for the invader.

If it's the kidney proteins that are confused with strep, about ten days after your sore throat begins you might begin swelling and passing urine that is dark and cloudy. You could end up with a serious kidney ailment. If it's the heart proteins that the antibodies attach to, then, about eighteen days after the strep throat, you'll get rheumatic fever, a serious heart and joint ailment. Rheumatic fever was thought to be a vanishing disease until 1987 when a series of outbreaks occurred. Outbreaks of rheumatic fever have occurred since that time on military bases, in suburban communities, and in the inner city. Although rheumatic fever is still a rare disease (in the United States—not so in the developing world), people need to keep their guard up and not let strep throat go untreated. The consequences can be too grave.

Do we need to run to the clinic to get checked every time we have a sore throat? After all, I've already told you that the vast majority of sore throats are not caused by strep. Actually, somewhere between 66 percent and 85 percent of the time, a sore throat will signal a viral infection. The problem is, you can't tell without being checked which sore throats require antibiotics and which can be ignored. You can't tell by looking, by your temperature, or by any other home method. So, most of the time, getting checked is the best policy. One exception applies, however: if your sore throat is clearly part of a cold—your nose becomes conspicuously congested simultaneously with your sore throat—you need not bother being checked for strep.

The health provider who examines you for strep throat can offer you several different options. He or she can (1) do a rapid strep test on a swab of your throat and have some information within minutes; (2) do the gold standard test, a throat culture, which will be read in one or two days; or (3) start or not start an antibiotic.

At first blush, a decision based on the rapid test seems most logical. The problem is that rapid strep tests are most reliable when they're positive. If your test is positive, you'll be right to start treatment. However, there are many false-negative test results, so often a culture is performed anyway. If you choose to delay treatment but the culture comes back showing that you really did have strep, you will still have time to start antibiotics and prevent nephritis and rheumatic fever. This is an acceptable approach. However, you've now missed a few days of antibiotics that would have made you feel better more quickly, you have bought an extra test that was useless to you, and you've been contagious for an additional two days or so.

Another approach (and one that I favor) is to just do the throat culture and start antibiotics promptly. I am especially likely to start antibiotics when there is fever, tender lymph nodes at the angle of the jaw, or pus on the tonsils. Then, if the culture shows no strep, antibiotics can be stopped.

When a throat culture (or a rapid strep test, for that matter) does show group A strep, it is important to complete a full course of treatment. If penicillin is used, it takes ten days to reliably clear that strep from your throat. After a few days, the throat no longer hurts; *finish the medicine anyway.* After you've been diagnosed and treated for strep, be sure to get any other household members with symptoms checked as well.

Under certain conditions it is wise to have all of the rest of the throats in the house checked automatically. Do this whenever strep throat has been a recurring problem in the household or whenever one of the serious strep complications has occurred. Only at these times is it of value to repeat the throat culture as a test of cure after a course of penicillin. Failures can be treated with penicillin again, but this time it is best augmented with rifampin, an antibiotic that gets high levels in the throat. Another antibiotic called clindamycin (Cleocin) can also clear hard-to-treat strep.

For some reason, some people, usually children, are plagued with frequent recurrences of pharyngitis. Why their immune system has opened up that particular door is unclear, but in this group, even surgery becomes a consideration. Tonsillectomy used to be a common medical practice, but it was clearly overdone in the past. There are, however, some times when it can help you.

A tonsillectomy (or tonsillectomy and adenoidectomy) is sometimes needed for refractory ear infections or for sleep apnea or loud snoring, and it can also help certain persons with recurring sore throats. Dr. Jack Paradise and colleagues at the Children's Hospital in Pittsburgh put this to the test. (Their work is described in the article by Randall, Parker, and Kennedy, listed in the bibliography.) They selected a group of people who suffered frequent repeats of sore throats associated with fever over

101°F, swollen glands, pus in the throat, and/or positive strep cultures (not just scratchy throats); the doctors did tonsillectomy on some of these patients and just observed others. Eighteen percent of those who had surgery still had two or more streptococcal throat infections in the following two years, but 54 percent of those without surgery did.

So, if repeated strep throats are a problem for you, tonsillectomy is an option that may help. But tonsillectomy is not a guaranteed cure and carries with it the risks of surgery, primarily bleeding and pain. The American Medical Association suggests that tonsillectomy be considered for persons who have four or more definite cases of pharyngitis in one year.

People who have rheumatic fever once are particularly prone to get it again. And if they do, the damage inflicted on their heart valves may be seriously compounded. They may end up needing their heart valves replaced. In order to avoid such complications, any child who ever had rheumatic fever should remain on penicillin on an ongoing basis. The penicillin (or erythromycin, for those allergic to penicillin) can be given as a pill twice daily or as an injection once a month. Adults are at considerably less risk than children for streptococcal pharyngitis. Most people over twenty years old who have not had a rheumatic attack for at least five years can stop penicillin prophylaxis. Exceptions are those adults with high risk of exposure to strep: parents of young children, teachers, physicians, other medical care workers, military recruits, and others who live in crowded conditions. These persons should continue their antibiotic prophylaxis indefinitely.

Mono

Mono, short for infectious mononucleosis, is just another kind of pharyngitis but with some unique twists. This type of pharyngitis is caused by the Epstein-Barr virus (EBV), and is the illness that some people—usually teenagers and young adults—get when they encounter EBV for the first time. In addition to pharyngitis, which may look no different from and is easily confused with strep throat, persons with mono tend to get large swollen glands in the neck and experience profound fatigue. They also have an increased number of lymphocytes in their blood that look like a cell called a monocyte, hence the name of the illness. Also, as opposed to most viral sore throats, which usually resolve in less than a week, this illness tends to last two or three weeks and may last four to six.

The funny thing about EBV is that if you get it early enough in life you don't get the illness we call mono and you very likely won't get sick at all. Most kids do pick it up at a young age—50 percent by age five. By adulthood, 90 to 95 percent of us have antibodies to EBV. That means that the majority of adults have already been exposed to EBV and are immune to it, whether or not they ever had mono.

EBV is not highly contagious. You have to have intimate contact to pass it on. People shed the virus in their saliva, so the term "kissing disease" has been aptly applied. Nevertheless, only one in twenty persons with mono really knows where it was picked up. The problem is that EBV is all around. After first getting mono, a person may continue to shed virus particles for years; adults checked at random have EBV in their saliva up to 20 percent of the time. So, I am pleased to tell you that you probably are already immune to EBV and do not have to be concerned about getting mono. It is also true that persons with mono need no special isolation. Unfortunately, should you happen not to be immune, there are no special precautions you can take to substantially reduce your risk.

In persons with an intact immune system, there is no chronic form of EBV and mono does not recur.

Strep bacteria that invade

In 1924, disaster struck the family of President Calvin Coolidge. Calvin, Jr., developed a blister while playing tennis with his brother on the White House courts. The injury became infected with *Streptococcus pyogenes*, which later invaded his bloodstream. The president's son died as a result of that infection, as did 72 percent of those similarly afflicted with streptococcal "blood poisoning" in that era.

Well, you say, before penicillin became available in 1943, of course we had nothing to stop invasive strep, but that kind of problem is of historical interest only. Why, then, did puppeteer Jim Henson die of streptococcal bacteremia in 1990? Mr. Henson contacted a physician on a Saturday, complaining of a flulike illness, and was treated with the usual flu remedies. He became sicker and was admitted to New York Hospital on the following Tuesday. There, he was found to have group A strep in his blood and he developed toxic shock syndrome as a result. He was given antibiotics, but died in twenty hours nonetheless.

On May 27, 1994, the Communicable Disease Surveillance Center in England reported on the group A streptococcal infections of six persons living in Gloucestershire; three died. Although it was known that invasive *Streptococcus pyogenes* infections seemed to have returned in 1987, the reports of these cases in the British tabloids made quite a stir and focused interest on this disease. Despite the implication that it is a new disease, it is not. However, it's back! Even though there is a resurgence, the infection is still rare. The Centers for Disease Control and Prevention (CDC) estimates ten to fifteen thousand cases occur in the United States annually. (Millions of us get strep throat every year.)

The link between some of the toxic and invasive strep germs common in the preantibiotic era and now lies in their chemical makeup and in the toxins they release, rather than anything humans do to prevent or treat them. Then and now, these virulent strains cause three types of illness: bloodborne infection (termed bacteremia and commonly called blood poisoning); deep skin infections (medically termed cellulitis or fasciitis, and recently given the sensationalist label "flesh-eating bacteria"); and toxic shock syndrome (previously thought to be caused only by staph germs). Certain strains of *Streptococcus pyogenes* have a particularly fuzzy, hairlike surface coating (the M1 protein) that makes the bacteria resistant to ingestion by white blood cells and allows them to multiply rapidly in human blood. If you pick up one of these, you very well may end up with a bloodstream infection.

Some other strains of strep can manufacture an enzyme called protease that can dissolve skin proteins. These strains may promote deep skin infections, or fasciitis. Yet other group A strep may elicit the same kind of toxins (erythrogenic toxins) that led to scarlet fever in years past. These strains can cause toxic shock syndrome: a diffuse red rash, low blood pressure, and dysfunction of multiple organs. Why have these virulent strains returned now? No one really knows.

Typically, these types of strep infections occur in adults. Half the time you never find how the strep first entered the body, but the infection does usually involve the skin and the tissues just below the skin. Taken together, this group of severe and invasive streptococcal infections are responsible for a high mortality rate. About one patient in three dies. However, with prompt diligent treatment, patients may do well.

I had an otherwise healthy thirty-six-year-old male patient who noted a blister on his thigh. His high fever and dizziness (due to low blood pressure) prompted him to come to the hospital right away. There, I found the blister to be the tip of an iceberg-shaped thigh infection. His blood culture grew the group A strep. With lots of penicillin and fairly extensive surgery he's pretty much back to normal.

Within a month after treating that case of invasive strep skin infection, I cared for a twenty-four-year-old woman who had given birth only three days earlier. She had been transferred from the maternity ward to the intensive care unit (ICU) because she had gone into shock and was covered with a sunburnlike rash. Group A grew from the vaginal secretions that are expected after delivery. She had all the signs of toxic shock syndrome. She spent only a few days in the ICU and recovered completely. (Her baby was fine.) It may be surprising, but almost a quarter of the time these serious strep infections are acquired in the hospital (see chapter 16).

In 1993 another patient of mine was not so lucky, although she's made it, too. This fifty-two-year-old woman had a gallbladder operation that went sour. After surgery, strep germs got into the wound and traveled under the skin all the way from just below the shoulder to just above the knee. This kind of galloping infection that spreads through the space between the skin and the muscle and destroys the body's tissues in its path is called necrotizing fasciitis. As is common to a lot of these cases, this patient had underlying medical problems to begin with (she was diabetic), and she was quite obese. After ten months and after multiple and extensive surgeries, she was able to leave the hospital and go to a rehabilitation center. She is still nearly bedridden, but is determined to recoup and walk back under her own power to thank the ICU staff.

What can we do to avoid these life-threatening strep infections? First of all, we need not live in constant fear. They are extremely rare. However, we must give prompt attention to skin infections like impetigo, wound infections, and to strep throat. And, when one person in a family contracts any of these severe strep infections, it is definitely worthwhile to check the rest of the household. In the early 1990s, Dr. Benjamin Schwartz and his co-workers at the CDC studied the spread of strep that caused invasive infections. They found twelve clusters of spread within families. The adults who picked it up tended to have the severe invasive disease, while the kids usually just carried the germ in their throat or had pharyngitis. In families (and in dorms, nursing homes, and the like) where a case of serious strep infection has occurred, each resident must have a throat culture. All strep found there must be eradicated.

3 *Urinary tract infections*

*T*his chapter is primarily for women. More than five million episodes of urinary tract infections (UTIs) occur annually in the United States, and the vast majority of them occur in women. About 3 percent of all women see the doctor each year for a UTI. At least one in five women will experience at least one UTI during her lifetime, and recurrences are not uncommon. Fortunately, for women, UTIs are not usually severe illnesses and are not an indication of a more serious underlying abnormality. But men, especially young men, get UTIs infrequently, and when a man gets a UTI, something else is wrong: a stone, an enlarged prostate, something.

Why the difference between the sexes? The most important reason seems to do with basic anatomy. The urethra, in both men and women, is the tube that connects the bladder with the outside world. The bladder is where most UTIs occur, and normally it is sterile. In men, the urethra is a generous 20 centimeters (about 8 inches) in length. For bacteria, it's a long swim up to the male bladder, and against the current. In women, the urethra is only 4 centimeters in length (only about an inch and a half). Also, UTIs occur when bacteria that normally inhabit the colon and get excreted in feces ascend the urethra. In women, the opening of the urethra is close to the rectum, and the warmth and moistness of the area provide conditions that are conducive to bacterial growth. Strategies to prevent UTIs are really only necessary and important for women.

Understanding how the UTI comes about helps you grasp and remember how preventive techniques work. The bacterium that causes over 95 percent of UTIs is *Escherichia coli*, or *E. coli* for short. While *E. coli* is one of the common bacteria in the colon, it is far from being the most common one there. The reason this germ has a penchant to get into the bladder is probably because it has molecules on its surface that stick to the cells lining the vagina and the urethra. The vagina, of course, is interposed between the rectum and the opening of the urethra. And that's how UTIs happen: *E. coli* or similar bacteria gain a foothold by colonizing the vagina, and then move to the cells around the urethra. If the chemical milieu there allows their survival, then the bacteria can either swim up the urethra (*E. coli* is motile) or be forced up mechanically, for example, during sex. Then, if the bladder is not too hostile an environment, they'll multiply there. When they reach significant numbers—over 100 bacteria per milliliter of urine (or about 5 per drop)—the body sends in white blood cells to fight back. Inflammation ensues. Now, the bladder lining gets irritated. It may even bleed and its muscle becomes irritable. So, the owner of that bladder experiences the urgent need to urinate frequently, pain on urination, and cloudy, possibly bloody or malodorous, urine.

There are a number of things that have definitely been associated with the development of UTIs in otherwise healthy women. These are sexual activity, the use of the diaphragm and spermicidal foam or jelly for contraception, and the changes that occur in women's vaginal membranes and secretions after menopause. (Oral contraceptive use, tampon use, the frequency of washing, and the direction a woman wipes herself after going to the bathroom have been shown *not* to be risk factors for UTI.) As you might predict, UTIs are most common in older women and after periods of increased sexual activity—"honeymoon cystitis" is real.

Of the known risk factors for UTI, sexual activity is most important. For example, the Student Health Service at the University of Pennsylvania compared the sexual history of female students with UTIs with those of students coming to the clinic for other reasons. The students diagnosed with a UTI were fifty-eight times more likely to have had sexual intercourse in the preceding forty-eight hours than the other students. In those women already colonized with *E. coli*, the mechanical aspects of sexual intercourse drive bacteria up into the urethra and bladder.

Fortunately, there are things you can do to diminish the risk of UTIs after sexual intercourse. The flushing action of urine as you empty your bladder is protective. So, urinate soon after sex. If you follow this practice and still find you are prone to UTIs after sex, antibiotics will work. Gatifloxacin (Tequin), ciprofloxacin (Cipro), and trimethroprim-sulfamethoxazole (Septra, Bactrim) are best for this purpose. (The latter, a sulfa drug, is the least expensive of the the three.)

Interestingly, a single antibiotic pill taken by mouth after sex will work. For example, in 1994 Drs. Alphonse Pfau and Theodore G. Sacks reported results of their study of a group of women prone to UTI. Thirty-three of these women had a combined total of 130 UTIs over an eight-month period. The doctors prescribed a single postsex antibiotic pill. Over the ensuing fifteen months, only one UTI occurred in the entire group.

Several medical studies have shown that women who use a diaphragm with a spermicide for contraception increase their risk of acquiring UTIs. We used to think that the physical effects of the diaphragm's ring was the culprit; that by putting direct pressure on the urethra it kinked the flow of urine and thereby promoted bladder infection. However, Drs. Raul Raz and Walter Stamm, at the University of Washington, have shown that, in students coming to their Student Health Center, users of condoms with spermicidal foam were just as much at risk of UTI as users of the diaphragm with spermicidal jelly.

It may be that the spermicide is the culprit. Spermicide is

actually a chemical called nonoxynol-9. It kills not only sperm, but certain bacteria as well. And, in the vagina, it will kill the normal inhabitants, primarily bacteria called lactobacilli. Spermicide does not kill *E. coli*, though, and may in some way promote its entry into the urethra. In any case, women who have a problem with UTIs should choose a contraceptive method that involves neither the diaphragm nor spermicidal jelly or foam.

UTIs are even more frequent in older women. Ten to 15 percent of women over age sixty will be plagued by frequent recurrences. In younger women, estrogens affect the vaginal secretions in such a way that lactobacilli are encouraged to grow. These bacteria produce lactic acid, which inhibits the growth of *E. coli* and other UTI-causing germs. In menopause, the ovaries stop producing estrogen, lactobacilli disappear, there is less acid in the vagina, and *E. coli* begins to grow there. This sets the stage for UTI in older women. But this situation can be reversed. If you replace the estrogen, the risk of UTI diminishes dramatically.

Vaginal estrogen can be replaced in one or both of two ways. You can apply vaginal cream, for example, estriol (Estrace), nightly for two weeks and then twice weekly, or you can take estrogen internally. Estrogen is available in pill, patch, and injectable forms. However, taken systemically, estrogen may promote cancer and blood clots in some women.

There is one other thing women who are particularly prone to UTIs can do: drink cranberry juice. It is an old folk remedy, but it can work. A team of researchers at Harvard put it to the test. In a group of women whose average age was seventy-eight, those who drank 300 milliliters (about 9 fluid ounces) of cranberry juice cocktail daily were 42 percent less likely to get a UTI than their counterparts who did not have the juice. Contrary to popular belief, though, the cranberry juice does not

---
TABLE 3.1
What women can do to prevent urinary tract infections

For all women:
❑ Urinate after sex.

For women who are prone to UTIs:
❑ Avoid using either a diaphragm or spermicide.
❑ Drink at least one tall glass of cranberry juice daily.
❑ Consider taking an antibiotic pill after sex.
❑ After menopause, consider replacement estrogens.

---

acidify the urine. Rather, it has chemical properties that interfere with the ability of *E. coli* to attach to cells.

Even if they follow all the rules (see table 3.1), some women still get UTI after UTI. These patients should ask their doctors about antimicrobial prophylaxis, the taking of a single antibiotic pill each night at bedtime until the period of susceptibility wanes. Such a program has helped many women get through a tough six or twelve months.

4 *Infections of the skin*

Of all your organs, your skin has the most contact with the germs surrounding you. It is your first and most important line of defense against infection. Therefore, we have evolved a number of mechanisms by which our skin protects us. It constitutes a physical barrier; it also secretes certain oils and maintains an acid-base balance that is repellent to harmful bacteria and fungi. Moreover, the skin is constantly replacing itself; you have a whole new layer every month. As the top layer of skin sloughs off, germs that may have built up there fall off with the old skin cells. We have also developed a symbiotic relationship with certain helpful bacteria that normally inhabit our skin and antagonize potentially injurious strains.

Although our skin is an efficient barrier, many things, most as mundane as insect bites, can breach it. So infections of our skin are very common. And the common bacterial germs described in other sections of this book, particularly *Staphylococcus aureus* and group A streptococci, are the biggest offenders. But, fungi are also common invaders of our skin (athlete's foot, for example). Viruses, although they develop inside the body rather than outside it (in forms like fever blisters and chickenpox), are common, too. Different approaches are needed to prevent common bacterial, fungal, and viral infections of the skin, so I'll analyze each of these groups separately.

Bacteria

There are a number of different forms of bacterial skin infections that are worth distinguishing. Impetigo is probably the commonest of them. It is caused by strep. Early on, it looks like a cluster of small pimples, but soon they rupture and are covered with a golden crust. Impetigo, like strep throat (see chapter 2), can lead to a kidney disease called poststreptococcal glomerulonephritis. Only certain strains of strep tend to cause this complication. If these strains are present in the community, you chance of getting kidney disease after impetigo can be as high as 2 to 5 percent. Sometimes *Staphylococcus aureus* causes impetigo, and in that case it might form a large blister. When an impetigo invasion goes deeper, the skin has a punched-out look and the infection is called ecthyma. Erysipelas is the name for a particular group A strep infection of the skin, usually on the face. It has been called "Saint Anthony's fire" because of its vivid red color and rapid onset and spread.

The rash called cellulitis occurs when staph or strep spread under large areas of the skin, usually on the shins, and is associated with fever and chills. Persons with diabetes and poor blood flow are particularly prone to this (see chapter 13). Hot-tub cellulitis is caused by a germ called *Pseudomonas aeruginosa* that loves to grow in hot, aerated water. Usually one to five days after exposure, it gives rise to small, very itchy pimples on areas that were submerged.

Furunculosis is the medical term for boils, which are abscesses of hair follicles caused by staph. They tend to occur on the nape of the neck, the face, buttocks, thighs, breasts, and armpits, but will not occur where there's no hair. When a group of boils coalesce into one larger and deeper structure, it is called a carbuncle.

Bacterial skin infections are very common around the fingernails and toenails. These areas commonly get rubbed and macerated, and the crevices on the sides of the nail are a fine environment for bacterial growth. Such an infection is termed paronychia, which just means "alongside the nail" in Greek. *Staphylococcus aureus* causes most paronychia.

Skin infections from animal bites are very common. It has been estimated that one of every two Americans will be bitten at some time by an animal or another person. There are between one and two million bites reported each year in the United States. Although the vast majority of them are minor or trivial, the remainder account for 1 percent of the visits people make to hospital emergency rooms. Of the animal bites that require medical treatment, 80 percent are dog bites, most often inflicted on men. Dog bites most commonly become infected with *Staphylococcus aureus*. Women tend to sustain cat bites more often than men do, and these wounds are more likely to become infected with a virulent germ called *Pasteurella multocida*. *Pasteurella* will produce obvious symptoms of infection in less than twelve hours.

Human bite wounds are the dirtiest of them all, because our mouths have high levels of bacteria—mostly the anaerobic kind that grow where the oxygen content is low. The "clenched fist injury" that occurs when a victim's teeth scrape the knuckle of an assaulter is an ironic form of retribution because it often produces a particularly bad infection that involves the bones and joints and requires surgery for repair.

So, what can we do to prevent this collection of unpleasantness? First of all, maintain ordinary good hygiene: bathe or shower once daily. This will help keep the number of pathogens low on your skin. If you are particularly prone to skin infections, occasionally using a germicidal soap such as one with triclosan (Dial) or chlorhexidine (Hibiclens) may also be worthwhile. Secondly, anytime you get a chink in your armor, any break in the skin, tend to it without delay. Persons who suffer recurrent boils are likely carrying high levels of staph in their nose; getting rid of those staph is discussed in chapter 16.

Cleaning wounds and bites correctly is very important. The most important part of that chore is purely mechanical. Physically flushing any contaminating bacteria or other foreign material out of a wound is essential. Any foreign material (gravel or splinters, for example) left in a wound markedly increases the chance of infection. This was demonstrated nicely in experiments in which a single stitch placed in an animal's skin promoted a staphylococcal infection with 10,000 fewer bacteria than would otherwise be needed. So, flush minor wounds with tap water and wash them out vigorously. If the wound is small enough, clean it with ordinary soap and water.

After a wound is cleaned, sterilize it. Many different preparations are available for doing this, but probably the best is povidone-iodine (Betadine). Keep some in the family medicine cabinet. Povidone-iodine solution does not sting, has excellent germicidal activity, and is a thin liquid so that it can easily be distributed to the recesses of the wound. If it is not used for a prolonged period, it doesn't injure the normal tissue, and few people are allergic to it. (Triple antibiotic ointments tend to just stay on the surface of a wound, and 6 to 8 percent of people can become allergic to the neomycin component in them.)

After painting the wound with a germicide, let it dry. Then cover the wound so that new germs won't get into it, using a bandage that breathes. Elevate any wounds that get swollen, because the serum that collects in an area of injury is a great culture medium for bacteria.

Few ordinary wounds, and many fewer of those treated as I have suggested, get infected. Bites are different, though, in that they have a higher rate of infection even if treated correctly. This is because more virulent germs are present in the mouths of dogs, cats, and humans than are present on the skin or in the environment, and these germs may be injected more deeply during the injury. Preventive antibiotics are often helpful after a bite wound. After certain bites, be sure to get started on antibiotics: those that are on the hand, that involve a joint, that are swollen, or that involve a deep puncture. The best advice is to seek medical attention promptly for all but trivial bites.

Fungi

The fungi that commonly infect our skin are called dermatophytes (from the Greek for "grows on skin"). These dermatophytes are fungi that thrive in the top, dead layer of our hair, nails, and skin. This layer contains a protein called keratin, fodder for dermatophytes. Most of us have had one or more fungus infections of our skin. Many of them are common, such as athlete's foot and ringworm. Athlete's food mostly infects men; one in ten men have it at any given time.

Doctors call these infections "tinea" and give each one a second Latin name according to where on the body the dermatophytes are growing: tinea pedis (athlete's foot), tinea cruris (jock itch), tinea capitis (scalp), tinea barbae (beard), tinea unguium (under the nails), and tinea corporis (ringworm—which is not caused by a worm at all).

Although dermatophyte fungi are all around us, they need help to get started growing under the skin. For example, if you immerse your perfectly intact foot in a solution teeming with dermatophytes, nothing happens. If you do the same thing with a minor cut in your skin, you will get tinea pedis.

Fungus infections of the skin are diseases of civilization. In cultures where barefootedness or sandals are the norm, people do not get athlete's foot. We get athlete's foot when we expose our feet to an appropriate fungus and then cover them with footwear that doesn't breathe. The spaces between our toes tend to become warm and wet. Not only does this provide the fungus with optimal conditions for growth, but it macerates the skin. The skin becomes soft and gets cracks in it—perfect places for the fungus to invade. In Vietnam, American soldiers spent days on end actively moving about while wearing army boots and fatigues in a hot, wet environment. They constantly became chafed. It is not surprising that they were plagued with tinea pedis, tinea corporis, and tinea cruris. In Vietnam, these were simply called "jungle rot."

How can you prevent fungal infections of your skin? You can do a few things to avoid the fungus in the first place, but mostly you need to keep the conditions on your skin unfavorable. Sometimes, a pet will carry fungal germs. Just be sure to keep hands off dogs or cats with skin infections and take them to their veterinarian promptly. But more often we encounter dermatophyte fungi in environments frequented by other people who are carrying these germs: gyms and health clubs, for example. In those places, avoid trafficked areas that are moist. More importantly, keep your skin dry and intact. Tight clothing and footwear should be avoided by anyone prone to dermatophytes. If you fit into that category, wear porous shoes and loose underwear, and shower frequently. If someone is particularly prone to fungi, applying an over-the-counter antifungal cream such as terbinafine (Lamisil) once or twice a week may be helpful as well.

Viruses

Don't be shocked, but you probably have herpes. Blood tests show that more than half of adult Americans do. But the most common type of herpes simplex virus (HSV) we carry is HSV-1, as opposed to HSV-2, the cause of genital herpes (see chapter 10). The type 1 virus is the cause of what is most commonly called a fever blister.

The typical sore caused by HSV-1 usually occurs on the outer portion of the lip, always somewhere around the mouth, and tends to recur. The first indication of it is usually burning, stinging, or itching, followed shortly thereafter by a small cluster of tiny blisters. When the blisters rupture, the infection tends to coalesce into an open sore. As it heals, it develops a honey-colored crust on its surface. It is usually better within a week and leaves no remnant after three weeks. Approximately one-quarter of us experience these annoyances repeatedly, generally in the same spot. Usually the recurrences happen no more than once yearly, but a small minority are inflicted with monthly fever blisters.

Unlike bacteria or fungi, when viruses infect our skin, they get there from inside our bodies. For example, we usually first pick up HSV-1 infection in childhood from close contact with our family. Anyone who has had HSV-1 in the past will excrete the virus intermittently in their saliva, whether or not they are having a fever blister at the time. When we first get HSV-1, there are usually no symptoms. However, if you get it for the first time as an adult, it can sometimes cause severe ulcers inside the mouth, not on the outer lip.

There really isn't much you can do to avoid the initial infection with HSV-1; just don't have direct contact with someone showing a fever blister, especially not with their mouth, if you've never had a fever blister yourself. Fever blisters, though—even the first one—are always recurrences. It works like this: After you have your first experience with the virus (which, again, you are usually not aware of) it migrates up through a nerve fiber. After it establishes itself in a nerve cell, it becomes dormant there. Later, some trigger, often unidentified, induces it to start growing again. Then, the virus will travel back down the nerve fiber and show up at the nerve's endings on the skin as a fever blister.

The trigger that incites HSV-1 to start growing again is often the same for any given individual. If you get fever blisters, you have to try to figure it out for yourself. Common provoking factors are exposure to sunlight (whether on the beach in summer or skiing in winter), menstrual periods, fever, and stress. Obviously, only one of these is easily controlled. If sun triggers fever blisters for you, you're lucky. You can simply apply sunscreen when needed to your lips and the other areas around your mouth. That works well. If you repeatedly and frequently get fever blisters following stimuli beyond your control, you could ask your physician to supply you with an antiherpes antibiotic to start whenever you know a fever blister is beginning. One is called acyclovir (Zovirax) and is best taken in pill form. If you are among the unfortunate ones who get very frequent recurrences, taking a small daily dose of acyclovir is something you might need to consider.

The other common viral infection of the skin is chickenpox, medically termed varicella. The virus that causes chickenpox is called varicella-zoster virus (VZV) because it is the cause of shingles (zoster) as well.

VZV first enters your body through the air. You breathe it in. It is highly contagious. In fact, if you've never had chickenpox, you have a 90 percent chance of acquiring it if someone in your household gets it. The infected person is contagious as much as two days before a rash appears, and for about four days after the rash appears. (School and work guidelines are conservative, though: you may return seven days after the rash appears or after all the sores are crusted.) You can also get chickenpox by contacting someone who has shingles, but you do not catch shingles from another person. Shingles occurs when your very own VZV, which has remained latent in your nerve cells (just as HSV does) ever since you had chickenpox, reactivates. Whereas chickenpox causes a rash of small blisters on a red base (like dewdrops on a rose petal) scattered anywhere and all over the entire body, shingles occurs only along the path of the nerve it reactivates from. So shingles is a discrete band of small blisters, always only on one side of the body.

Chickenpox is generally a benign disease that, prior to common use of varicella vaccine, 3.7 million Americans got every year. There were about 9,000 hospitalizations because of it. If you don't catch chickenpox when you are a kid, it can be more serious in adulthood. It is a particular concern for pregnant women (see chapter 15) and for anyone whose immune system is compromised (see chapter 14), but any adult with chickenpox is likely to have a more severe case than a child has, and in adults, pneumonia may result.

If you are an adult who has never had chickenpox, you need to take every precaution to avoid catching it. If you can, avoid being in the same room with a person who has chickenpox. Also, because the virus can travel along air currents, even being on the same floor with an infected person may be a hazard. The virus can *linger* in the air, too; it has been detected hours after a contagious person has left the room. It is often difficult, though, for you to avoid a person with chickenpox, as when it is your own child. The bright side of that dilemma is that as many as 80 percent of adults who don't think they've had chickenpox actually really did and are immune. If you need to find out, you can get a blood test done to check your immune status.

The whole problem with chickenpox in the United States may be nearing an end. On March 17, 1995, after two years of deliberation, the Food and Drug Administration (FDA) finally approved a chickenpox vaccine. Many had been awaiting the vaccine because it had been used in Japan for years. It was first developed there at Osaka University in 1974, and it was licensed in 1989 in Japan and Korea, where millions of doses have been administered. The concerns in the United States about this vaccine were twofold: First, since it is a live vaccine, would it come back as shingles? And if so, would shingles be very common or very severe? Well, as it turns out, shingles occurs at a much lower rate in individuals who have been vaccinated than in the individuals who've had natural chickenpox, and it tends not to be severe. The second concern was whether the protective immunity of the vaccination would wear off as people grow older. If so, this would shift the disease to adults, in whom the disease tends to be severe. We now know, though, that the vaccine confers immunity that lasts at least eleven years, and the Merck Company has agreed to monitor a group of persons who have received it to determine when (or if) booster shots might be required in the future.

This new vaccine is called Varivax and is given by injection. Children aged twelve months to twelve years will receive a single injection, given at the same time as the measles-mumps-rubella vaccine (MMR). Those thirteen years old and older need two injections given one or two months apart. After vaccination, some individuals (about 5 percent) get a mild rash. A sore, red arm is the most common side effect (25 percent), and fever may also occur (10 percent). The vaccine is 95 percent effective in healthy children. When it fails, the cases of chickenpox recipients get are generally very mild.

It is intended that all children will receive the chickenpox vaccine. As the few adults who get chickenpox usually get it after exposure to kids, the risk to adults will drop off dramatically. However, some adults may still want to receive the vaccine, although in them it is only 70 percent effective. If you are an adolescent or adult and you've never had chickenpox (or you're not sure), you may want to get your blood tested to see if you're already immune. If you are, that immunity, which you got naturally, will last for the rest of your life. If you are not immune to chickenpox, there are certain situations in which getting the vaccine will be an important thing to do: if you work with small children, if you are in contact with other persons whose immune systems are poor, if you are a woman of childbearing age (but not pregnant), or if you've been exposed to chickenpox in the prior three days.

Two

Infections you get from your environment

5 *Lyme disease and tickborne infections*

Lyme disease strikes fear in many Americans, and yet, no one dies of Lyme. It may be so scary because it afflicts the unsuspecting and because it can be crippling. You can pick up Lyme disease and not know it, and, once you're ill, it is sometimes hard for doctors to diagnose or treat. With a bit of care, you can avoid Lyme disease in the first place.

Lyme disease is an infection caused by a spiral-shaped bacterium, or spirochete, called *Borrelia burgdorferi*. Although the manifestations of Lyme disease can vary widely from person to person, it does follow a basic pattern. A typical case of Lyme disease starts at the site of a tick bite. There, in less than a month, an expanding red rash often develops. It becomes ring- or target-shaped and the size of an adult's open hand. This rash is called erythema chronicum migrans (or ECM), and it vanishes on its own in days to months. ECM may be associated with flulike symptoms which indicate that the spirochetes are now circulating through the bloodstream and infecting other areas of the body.

Most patients, if untreated, will get arthritis weeks to years after ECM fades. The knees are most commonly affected. The arthritis is usually episodic, but in 10 percent of those infected it becomes chronic and permanently debilitating.

Lyme disease may also affect the nervous system. The range of neurological abnormalities is protean. An inflammation of the membranes over the brain (a mild form of meningitis) can occur and cause a headache and a stiff neck. Individual nerves may also be affected, often those going to the face. The muscles they serve may weaken; for example, a facial droop may occur (often called Bell's palsy). Lyme disease can also slow the heartbeat and weaken the heart muscle, and it is a newly recognized cause of miscarriage and birth defects. Especially when treated late, Lyme disease can also cause chronic fatigue, but not usually without some other aspects of the disease as well.

Is Lyme disease preventable? Yes. Lyme disease occurs after the bite of a tick. No tick bite, no Lyme. But the risk for Lyme disease varies with season, location, and the type of ticks you encounter. Let me explain further.

As with most infections, your primary weapon in prevention is knowledge. For Lyme disease it is understanding the spirochete's life cycle (see figure 5.1). A common field mouse and the Lyme disease spirochete have a sort of nonaggression pact. The mouse carries the microorganism in its bloodstream and both parties remain unhurt. (In fact, most wild animals are uninjured by this germ, while most domestic animals come down with the disease.) The mouse that carries it in the environment is the white-footed mouse.

The white-footed mouse is an easy target for ticks. A particular tick, the tiny deer tick (also called the black-legged tick), makes a living feeding off the blood of the white-footed mouse. The deer tick prefers this field mouse to all other sources of fresh blood. If the field mouse is infected with the spirochete, the tick becomes infected as well. The Lyme disease spirochetes then survive happily in the gut of the tick. Moreover, when the tick feeds on an uninfected mouse, the tick regurgitates the spirochete into the bloodstream of the mouse; the circle is closed and the life cycle of *B. burgdorferi* goes on. So how do people become involved in this tidy scheme? Actually, to our misfortune, we interfere in it.

Ticks mature in discrete stages. In autumn, the adult deer tick (whose scientific name is *Ixodes scapularis*, formerly named *Ixodes dammini*) feeds, just once. It can feed on any number of

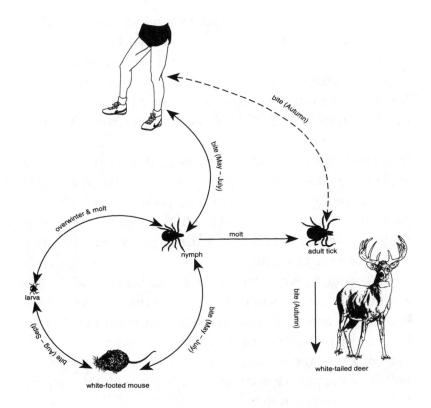

FIGURE 5.1 *The life cycle of the Lyme disease agent*
The Lyme disease agent continues a natural cycle in nature. Man intrudes.

different animals, but it relishes the white-tailed deer. Only in areas where deer are abundant are deer ticks found in substantial numbers. The deer seems critical to the survival of deer ticks. Generally, though, humans don't get Lyme disease from the adult ticks (and deer themselves are not a risk to us at all). We are more prone to encounter young ticks. After the adult female feeds, she lays eggs from which larvae hatch. Larvae molt and become nymphs in the spring. In the usual course of nature, a nymph will take its blood meal in May, June, or July, and it seeks the white-footed mouse. Here comes the people part.

It's spring, and the poppy-seed-sized nymph is poised on low vegetation awaiting a mouse. Unfortunately, it is not very discriminating. A person will do nicely. When a human foot brushes this blade of grass, the nymph attacks and feeds for a few days. The bite is painless and often unnoticed. It is the nymph form of the deer tick that most often transmits *B. burgdorferi* spirochetes to humans to cause Lyme disease. Less frequently, adult ticks infect humans as well. As you recall, in autumn the adult female deer tick (now the size of an apple seed) can be found on grass or brush, poised at knee height in hopes of a deer passing by. She will feed on a large mammal for over a week, more noticeably than a nymph but also painlessly and with little itch.

As you might expect from knowing the life cycle of the tick and the habits of human beings, most cases of Lyme disease begin in the months of June and July. This is the time to take most precautionary measures. However, as long as there are ticks of any stage feeding, transmission is possible. In the United States, this can occur anytime from the first day of May to the last day of November.

Lyme disease has been found worldwide, but only in those areas with the right mix of infected rodents, ticks, and deer, all in proximity to humans. In the United States it occurs primarily in three areas: the Northeast (especially coastal areas), north central (particularly in Wisconsin and Minnesota), and the Pacific Coast (especially northern California). There are fourteen states in which Lyme disease is not uncommon. These are listed for you in table 5.1.

Diseased ticks can be carried into other states by birds and, as the deer population expands, new areas are becoming involved. But certain areas remain notorious for Lyme. The disease was discovered in Lyme, Connecticut, and this rural community continues to have the highest rate of infection in

TABLE 5.1
Where Lyme disease is found

States in which Lyme disease is common[a]

Northeast	North Central	Pacific
Connecticut	Minnesota	California
Delaware	Wisconsin	
Maine		
Maryland		
Massachusetts		
New Hampshire		
New Jersey		
New York		
Pennsylvania		
Rhode Island		
Virginia		

Other states where it can also be found, but less often

Alabama	Louisiana	South Carolina
Arizona	Michigan	Tennessee
Arkansas	Missouri	Texas
Florida	Nebraska	Utah
Idaho	Nevada	Vermont
Illinois	New Mexico	Washington
Indiana	North Carolina	West Virginia
Iowa	North Dakota	Wyoming
Kansas	Ohio	
Kentucky	Oregon	

SOURCE: Centers for Disease Control and Prevention (CDC), "Final 2002 Reports of Notifiable Diseases," *Morbidity and Mortality Weekly Report* 52 (2003): 741–750.
[a]In each of these states, over 100 cases were reported in 2002.

the country. However, where the human population density is greater and conditions for transmission also exist, there are bound to be more cases. In fact, two New York counties, Westchester and Suffolk, account for over 40 percent of all U.S. cases of Lyme disease. Other areas in which outbreaks have occurred include Shelter Island and Fire Island in New York, and Ipswich, Cape Cod, and Great Island in Massachusetts.

Avoiding tick bites

If you avoid tick habitats altogether, you will never get Lyme disease. But you would have to exclude all contact with our natural environment. For me, that is much too dear a price to pay. In addition, many people's occupations put them at risk for tick bite; for example, linesmen, surveyors, landscapers, and park rangers. Three basic kinds of precautions can make venturing out into grassy, brushy, and forested areas quite safe, however: (1) denying ticks access to your skin, (2) repelling ticks, and (3) removing ticks.

If you go trekking in tick country, wear long pants. They do not have to be heavy; in fact, a loose fit is better. The ticks are usually on grass or brush, so there should be no break between pants and socks. You might tuck your pants inside your socks or boots, or put a loose rubber band or masking tape over your pant legs. If you lie down, cover your neck and head as well.

Insect repellents will help keep ticks off your skin, but as anyone who has gone outdoors on a summer evening knows, they are hardly foolproof. To get the best results, pick a repellent with DEET (*N,N*-diethyl-3-methylbenzamide) as its active ingredient. The optimal concentration of DEET is unknown but the pure (actually, 95 percent) stuff on the market is overkill and could be dangerous. Around 30 percent may be better; several popular brands have that concentration. DEET can be absorbed through the skin and has caused dermatitis and allergies. In excessive amounts it can also be toxic to the nervous system. Follow directions and consider reapplying after swimming, washing, or sweating. Keep DEET away from eyes, nose, mouth, and open wounds. Be particularly careful using it on children.

It may be very helpful to use a strong repellent on your clothes. Choose one with permethrin (or pyrethrin). For those who enjoy leaving all civilization back at the trail head, these last on your clothes for over a week if properly applied. Treat your dog as well: your veterinarian or pet store can supply an acaricide, a spray or powder that kills ticks and mites.

If you've applied appropriate repellents and worn appropriate clothes, you have lessened your chances of getting tick bites, but they can still occur. You will still need to check thoroughly for ticks on your person. Here's why. It takes time for the tick to transmit Lyme disease. When shorn sheep were subjected to infected ticks, no sheep became infected when the ticks were removed before twenty-four hours had gone by. If the ticks were allowed to cling for a second day, there was a 50 percent chance of the sheep becoming infected. After day three, infection was universal. So, even if the ticks slip through your armor, if you look yourself (and the kids) over for ticks twice a day, you're unlikely to give them enough time to transmit infection to you. You won't be able to see certain places on your own body. The back of the head is one example. Get family or friends to help search there and return the favor.

Tick-bit! What to do?

It is disconcerting enough just to see that blood-engorged parasite burrowed deeply in your skin. Thought of later becoming ill with an infectious disease is even worse. Your basic instinct is to pinch it, pull it, toss it, and expect the worst. This is the natural response, but wholly inappropriate. Actually, your chance of having contracted an illness is small, even in endemic areas. In the areas where Lyme disease is most prevalent, about 1 percent of deer tick larvae, 25 percent of the nymphs, and 50 percent of the adults are infected with the Lyme spirochete, and bites of infected ticks transmit the disease only about 10 percent of the time; thus, fewer than 5 percent of deer tick bites in highly endemic areas result in disease. Nevertheless, to decrease that risk, do not panic. Instead: (1) Remove the tick gingerly, as I will describe, (2) try to generally identify it, and (3) in certain circumstances call your physician for antibiotics as an additional preventive measure.

There are countless folk methods for removing ticks. Well-meaning people are generally eager to give advice on their favorite technique. When scientifically scrutinized, though, most of these methods are wrong. Dr. Glen Needham of Ohio State University subjected five commonly recommended techniques to laboratory tests. He smothered ticks with petroleum jelly, painted them with fingernail polish, doused them with alcohol, and burned them with a hot match head. The object, of course, was to induce the tick to detach itself. The professor waited twenty-four hours for the ticks to disengage after each procedure and none did. The experiments showed that a tick does not crawl away if it is covered with goo or can't even move its legs. Moreover, heat will induce a tick to salivate and regurgitate, which may increase the chances of transmitting the disease to you. Worse, an engorged tick could burst and expose you to its infected body fluids.

Here is Dr. Needham's laboratory-proven procedure for tick removal. It extracted the intact parasite, including burrowed mouthparts, every time.

1. Use tweezers or blunt curved forceps, if available. If fingers are used, shield them with tissue, paper towel, or rubber gloves. (You can become infected from ticks by handling them.)

2. Grasp the tick as close to the skin surface as possible and pull upward with steady, even pressure. Do not twist or jerk the tick as this may cause the mouthparts to break off.

3. Take care not to squeeze, crush, or puncture the body of the tick as its fluids may contain infective agents.

4. Save the tick for later identification if you can. Place it in a closed container, preferably immersed in alcohol. Flushing the tick down the toilet is a good method ultimately to get rid of it.

5. Thoroughly disinfect the bite site with alcohol or another antiseptic and wash your hands with soap and water.

Lyme disease is the most common disease you get from ticks in the United States, but it is by no means the only one. If you get some idea of what kind of tick you've been exposed to, you can figure out what infections you might be at risk for. I cannot make you a tick expert, for I am not one myself, but the following is enough to help you get started at finding out what you need to know.

Ticks are oval. Although they look like insects, their bodies do not have segments. Four pairs of legs (only three pairs on larvae) and a beak (mouthparts) project from the oval.

Ticks come in only two basic families, soft ticks and hard ticks. The soft ticks are leathery, and can be readily identified because their mouthparts are hidden by their back when viewed from above. The soft-bodied ticks will transmit only one human disease in the United States, relapsing fever, and this only in very limited areas. The hard-bodied ticks are much more important vectors. The deer tick is a hard tick. So are the dog tick and the wood tick, both of which carry Rocky Mountain spotted fever.

As described above, deer ticks are small (see figure 5.2). From the tip of its pincerlike beak to the most posterior aspect of its body, and adult male *Ixodes scapularis* is a mere three millimeters (about one-eighth of an inch). Adult females and nymphs are progressively smaller, and the larvae are nearly microscopic. The backs of deer ticks are more lightly shaded toward the rear, the adult with an orange-red crescent. By comparison, dog ticks and wood ticks are about twice as large as deer ticks and have a lighter crescent toward their front.

If you do indeed remove a tick and believe it is the deer tick, should you take antibiotics to prevent Lyme disease? The answer is not entirely clear cut, but if you are in a high-risk area, it is yes. The answer is not clear because, though your chances of contracting Lyme disease from a given bite are quite small, the antibiotics given are really not very toxic, anyway. In areas of high risk in the Northeast, the actual chance of contracting Lyme disease following a tick bite is about 1 to 5 percent, and prophylactic antibiotics may be worthwhile. For several reasons, transmission in the Pacific states is much less efficient, and prophylactic antibiotics are probably unnecessary. Antibiotics are also not recommended to prevent any of the other tickborne illnesses, only to treat them.

Is it acceptable to simply wait and see if a rash develops? After all, ECM is quite a characteristic outbreak. The answer is no because 20 to 40 percent of people never have (or never recognize) ECM. If you miss ECM, a more serious problem in the joints, heart, or nervous system might be the first indication of Lyme disease. Intravenous treatment might become necessary or, worse, a complete cure might not be accomplished.

Call your doctor. He or she should go over the details of exposure with you, review your medical history, and discuss potential side effects of the medicine. The antibiotic that's usu-

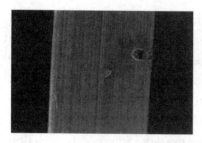 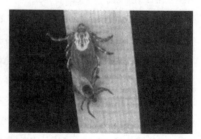

FIGURE 5.2 *Germ-carrying ticks*
A. The nymph form of the deer tick (*Ixodes scapularis*), shown on a blade of grass, is commonly found in spring. **B.** The adult female deer tick, found on taller vegetation, with the much larger dog tick (*Dermacentor variabilis*) for comparison.

Source: F. Matuschka and A. Spielman, "Images in Clinical Medicine," *New England Journal of Medicine* 327 (1992): 542. Reprinted by permission of the New England Journal of Medicine. Copyright 1992 Massachusetts Medical Society.

ally prescribed for a potential Lyme disease exposure is a tetracycline called doxycycline. It is the most effective antibiotic in pill form for killing *Borrelia burgdorferi.* The medicine is taken twice daily for fourteen days. Reactions are unusual but can include minor symptoms such as nausea, vomiting, allergies, and vaginitis, and doxycycline may magnify your usual propensity to sunburn. If doxycycline sits too long in your esophagus it may cause an ulcer, so don't take it just before you lie down at night, and wash it down well. Serious side effects to doxycycline are rare (about 0.01 percent). Do not take doxycycline (or any tetracycline) if you might be pregnant or if you are nursing. Tetracyclines are not given to children under eight years old (for one thing, they can stain growing teeth). Penicillin or erythromycin can be used as alternatives to tetracycline when it is not allowed.

One might ask, if antibiotics are available after the fact, why go to any effort to avoid tick bites? First, tick bites are painless and unless you are looking for them, they could go unrecognized. Furthermore, antibiotics do not eliminate all risk of Lyme disease, and antibiotics won't ward off many other diseases that are transmitted by ticks.

Lyme disease might be the most common disease carried by ticks, but it is not the most serious. Each season there are deaths from Rocky Mountain spotted fever. Several other tickborne diseases, although rare, can also be fatal. If you're careful about ticks, hoping to prevent Lyme disease, you can prevent these others simultaneously. Following is a list of the other tickborne infections in the United States, indicating how they could affect you, the tick that carries them, and where they are found.

❏ *Rocky Mountain Spotted Fever.* Carried by the dog tick and the wood tick (hard ticks). Initial fever, headache, and later, rash. Despite the name, found widely; mostly in Southeast, especially the Carolinas, and parts of the Midwest, especially Missouri and Oklahoma.

❑ *Ehrlichiosis.* Carried by hard ticks. Fever, headache, muscle aches; low blood counts; but rash occurs in less than a third of cases. Found in the Southeast and southern Midwest, especially Oklahoma, Missouri, and Arkansas.

❑ *Babesiosis.* Carried by *Ixodes*, the same kind of ticks that carry Lyme disease. Fever, chills, and muscle aches; if your spleen has been removed, more severe illness may occur. Found on the islands off the Northeast coast.

❑ *Colorado Tick Fever.* Carried by the larger hard ticks. Fever, headache, nausea, vomiting, eye pain, and aversion to light. Found in the mountainous areas of the western United States and Canada.

❑ *Tickborne Relapsing Fever.* Carried by soft ticks. Cycles of fever and nonfever lasting days at a time. Found in cabins infested with rodents in the mountains of California and Arizona.

❑ *Tick Paralysis.* Carried by various hard ticks. Weakness, followed by paralysis, progressing from the feet up, until the tick is found and removed. Found sparsely but widely across North America; a more severe form exists in Australia.

❑ *Tularemia.* Carried by various hard ticks. The bite site forms a tender black crust and the lymph glands swell; most common in the groin; high fever. Found in all fifty states, but especially South Central states such as Missouri, Arkansas, and Oklahoma.

Perhaps some of the anxiety about Lyme disease and about ticks has been exaggerated. Some people who have had only minimal exposure to ticks have become overly concerned. Having no reliable blood test to confirm or disprove suspected cases hasn't helped matters. Despite the confusion about Lyme disease, don't be confused about this. In the right environment, it's out there, and you need to take care.

6   *Food poisoning*

I love to hike and climb, to sail and canoe. So, when I lead trips for the Boy Scouts, I am not altogether altruistic. Therefore, it was with some element of guilt that I attended the yearly banquet honoring Scout leaders. The banquet is a special occasion and this year we dined on exceptional barbecue, prepared by a well-known caterer out in the countryside, a two-hour drive south of the city. The barbecue was delicious, the attendees received appropriate certificates, and we went home happy. I awoke at about three the next morning in a pool of sweat, and bolted for the bathroom. Dysentery went on for almost two days. I found out later that nearly all of the seventy attendees had experienced variations on the same theme. Two elderly leaders were hospitalized and we were all thankful it had not been a feast for the boys.

On the night of this outbreak I broke some of my own rules. I should have known better. I knew that chicken, beef, and pork not uncommonly come contaminated with *Salmonella* and must be handled appropriately. I should have realized that the meat had probably been kept at the temperature of a warm bath during the drive from the barbecue mecca to our banquet, and then allowed to sit even longer while dishes were finished and served. These are perfect growing conditions for bacteria. Indeed, my stool cultures were teeming with *Salmonella*. There are over fifty *Salmonella* outbreaks like ours yearly in the United States, and millions more cases occurring singly. We all survived our ordeal, but five thousand Americans die each year from foodborne infections.

Perhaps we don't respect food poisoning enough to take the care we should be taking to prevent it. I think many believe that since our species survived for so many years before we had potable water, sewage systems, or refrigeration, and long before there was a Food and Drug Administration or U.S. Department of Agriculture, food poisoning can't be a very serious problem. Yes, our species has survived, but lots of people have died along the way and many more have become very sick from contaminated food. Take, for example, Bangladesh, a virtual laboratory of enteric diseases for medical researchers. There, without the benefit of Western sanitation systems, diarrhea is a constant serious threat, killing many thousands yearly, usually the very young and the very old. Even if you were to move to Mexico and live there permanently, you would have a fifty-fifty chance of getting diarrhea every month. In the United States, despite relatively careful attention to sanitation, food preservation, and hygiene, foodborne diseases strike about seventy-six million people yearly.

The number of victims doesn't have to be that high. Following some simple rules will eliminate most food poisonings. That is what this chapter is about. Until regulatory agencies do a better job preventing contamination of food at its source and implement systems such as food irradiation and more sophisticated water purification, we will remain at risk for food poisoning.

Food-related illnesses can generally be divided into three categories. Actual food poisoning occurs when a toxin is already formed in the food before you eat it. This toxin is usually the by-product of bacteria that had contaminated the food. Botulism is a prime example. However, the most common type of food-related illness in industrialized countries is simple gastroenteritis. Gastroenteritis occurs when something you eat or drink is a vehicle for bacteria or viruses that subsequently grow in your bowels and cause an infection. It is generally manifested by fever, chills, sweats, nausea, vomiting, and diarrhea. My *Salmonella* illness was this type. Lastly, many parasites gain entry into your body in what you eat. Most parasites are fairly rare in North America, but we'll discuss a few that are common.

Certain foods are notorious for conveying particular food-related illnesses. Thus a practical way to classify such illnesses is by category of foodstuffs. Groupings of this kind are also a convenient way for me to warn you how not to get infected, as each class of food has its own set of rules. Before attacking this problem, one course at a time, there are a few general guidelines that apply to preventing all intestinal infections and poisonings.

This is a miracle age of medicine. Drugs cure and control many illnesses now that were the rampant scourges of the past. So it's not surprising that doctors and patients look to medications to help any health problem. However, medicines may now be overused. It is estimated that half our antibiotics are taken either unnecessarily or incorrectly. Many people seem to down Maalox, Tagamet, or other antacid drugs constantly. Both antibiotics and antacids can predispose you to intestinal infections. Take them only when you really need them.

The colon is normally filled with helpful bacteria, one trillion per gram of stool. These bacteria, among other things, don't allow room for harmful organisms to grow. When you take antibiotics to kill offending germs, you will kill many of the normal bacteria and may make yourself more susceptible to a bowel infection. For example, in outbreaks of dysentery due to *Salmonella*, persons taking antibiotics beforehand are more likely to come down with it than others who were equally exposed and not taking antibiotics.

Persons taking antibiotics often have soft stools and sometimes frank diarrhea (that is, liquid bowel movements). In a few cases, a particular and more serious infection called pseudomembranous colitis results. It is caused by a bacterium,

Clostridium difficile, which is resistant to many antibiotics. With the other bacteria diminished, it has a chance to overgrow in your colon. Worse yet, it releases a toxin that burns the colon lining; that leads to more diarrhea, cramps, and fever. This infection can be fatal. If you get diarrhea after antibiotics—it usually happens only two days after, but can happen up to six weeks later—you may need specific treatment with an additional antibiotic—metronidazole or vancomycin—to kill *Clostridium difficile*. For the next six months, you will need to avoid taking antibiotics. As always, take them only when you really need them.

Your most important defense mechanisms against infections are the barriers between your body and the outside environment. Your skin is the biggest one. Another is the muscles that seal your urinary tract unless you are emptying your bladder. And there is a complicated system of barriers in the respiratory tract, discussed in chapter 8. In the stomach, acid acts as your shield. Under ordinary conditions there, 99.9 percent of ingested bacteria are killed in thirty minutes. Normally, you have to ingest about one million bacteria to get typhoid fever or other *Salmonella* infections, but if your stomach acid is neutralized, only one thousand of the bacteria will do it. That's why you should take antacids or antacid medications only when really needed.

Vigilance in ensuring careful food handling could be much improved in the United States. Rules and regulations abound, but are often unenforced. Restaurants with violations of food-handling laws are ten times more likely to cause outbreaks of food poisoning than those that pass inspection. So, if you have heard of a restaurant that might have less than optimal food-handling technics, don't go there. If you know of someone who thinks they became ill at a particular establishment, believe them. Whatever the shortcomings in preventing food poisoning are in North America, they're worse in the nonindustrialized nations of the world. When traveling to these areas, follow the "cardinal rules for eating abroad" listed in table 7.1.

Some of you reading this chapter will be more susceptible to enteric infections than others. You must take extra care. I've already pointed out that neutralizing your stomach acid eliminates a major barrier to enteric infection. If you have chronic gastritis, if you have had surgery for ulcers, or if you have an HIV infection, you may have a medical condition called *achlorhydria*, which means "lack of stomach acid." HIV-infected persons are prone to diarrhea for many other reasons as well, and I discuss this in chapter 14. Persons with liver disease should pay particular attention to what they eat, too. Blood from the gut may be contaminated with bacteria that have passed through the intestinal membranes. This blood goes through the liver before reaching the rest of the body. During that passage, special cells in the liver filter out the unwanted microbes. If the liver is scarred, blood is diverted and this sieve function is bypassed.

Meat, poultry, and eggs

The U.S. Department of Agriculture categorizes all foods of animal origin as hazardous. They're right. To stick with the *Salmonella* example, this bacterium is a normal resident in the colon of most animals, including cows, pigs, and chickens. Not uncommonly then, our food sources become contaminated with *Salmonella*. Eggs often carry this bacterium, and often *Salmonella* infections are due to ingestion of foods made with grade A eggs. (Hens lay eggs through their vent, an exit shared by their intestines.)

Salmonella is not the only germ we get from animal food sources. The most common bacterium causing dysentery in Americans is called *Campylobacter*, and most of the time we get it from contaminated poultry. "Campy" can be cultured from over half of the chicken meat in processing plants and in a quarter of what is for sale in the market.

Escherichia coli (*E. coli* for short) is another colonic germ presenting a risk to meat eaters. You may remember news stories from 1993 telling of several people dying from contaminated, undercooked hamburgers in the state of Washington. They had ingested a bacterium designated *E. coli* 0157:H7. This organism can cause more than just gastroenteritis when it liberates a toxin (called verotoxin). When this toxin enters the circulation, serious bleeding disorders and kidney failure can ensue (called the hemolytic uremic syndrome).

As it turns out, you can find *E. coli* 0157:H7 in 1.5 to 3.5 percent of all ground beef, pork, poultry, and lamb. Dairy cattle, especially young animals, often carry it, so raw (unpasteurized) milk is another source of this disease. *Salmonella, Campylobacter*, and *E. coli* may be the most prominent bugs carried in foods we get from animals, but they are not alone. Table 6.1 gives you a more complete list.

So how can you protect yourself from gastrointestinal infections carried in meat, poultry, eggs, and dairy products? Heat and cold are your best defenses. Heat kills germs, and cold prevents them from multiplying. Heat will also inactivate many potent bacterial toxins like the verotoxin of *E. coli* and *botulinum*, the cause of botulism. Often, meat is already contaminated when we get it. *Bacillus cereus* and *Clostridium perfringens*, for example, are ubiquitous in meats. So cooking and cooling are the methods you must fall back on to keep bacteria at safe levels.

A common theme in food poisonings is, in fact, that food has been sitting at room temperature for too long. I call this temperature abuse. People often commit temperature abuse around holidays. At these times especially, foods (and the leftovers) tend to be left out during prolonged feasts. As a consequence, every year after Thanksgiving a number of people get

TABLE 6.1
Causes of food poisoning from animal sources

Causative agent	Most common food	Dishes that have caused outbreaks
Bacillus cereus	Pork	Barbecued chicken Barbecued pork Boiled beef Fried rice Sausage
Campylobacter jejuni	Poultry	Beef Chicken Cornish hen Goat's milk Raw milk
Clostridium botulinum	Varied	Venison jerky
Clostridium perfringens	Beef	Chicken Corned beef Turkey
E. coli 0157:H7	Beef	Hamburgers Raw milk Semisoft cheese Unpasteurized juice
Listeria monocytogenes	Dairy	Cottage cheese Ice cream Pork tongue Raw milk Soft cheese
Salmonella enteritidis	Eggs	Barbecue Eggnog Hollandaise Homemade ice cream Infant formula Powdered milk Raw milk Yogurt
Staphylococcus aureus	Varied	Corned beef Ham Raw milk
Trichinella spiralis	Pork	Bear meat Homemade sausage
Yersinia enterocolitica	Pork	Chitterlings Chocolate milk Pasteurized milk Raw milk Sausage

Salmonella food poisoning. One year after St. Patrick's Day, groups of celebrators in Ohio and Virginia got *Clostridium perfringens* diarrhea from corned beef.

Failure to properly control food temperature is the single most common mistake leading to food poisoning. Bacteria can multiply rapidly; some kinds can double their numbers every twenty minutes. But they can do this only in temperatures between 40° and 140°F (4.4° to 60°C). The National Restaurant Foundation calls this the "temperature danger zone" and instructs its members to keep all potentially hazardous foods out of this temperature range (see figure 6.1). But during food preparation, serving, and eating, this may not be possible. Add up in your mind the total accumulated time potentially hazardous foods spend in the danger zone. Four hours is too long. But since all food spends some time in the danger zone before you obtain it, allow only one hour of which you're aware. Over that, discard the meal.

If you really want to invite trouble, you'll eat meat or dairy products that haven't been cooked at all. Steak tartare may be a delicacy to some but it is lunacy to me. Eating raw eggs is also risky; you're apt to encounter them in Caesar salad, homemade eggnog and mayonnaise, undercooked French toast, eggs Benedict, hollandaise sauce, and meringue. Even partly cooked eggs can still have live *Salmonella* in them. Dr. T. J. Humphrey and his colleagues in Britain's Public Health Laboratory purposely contaminated some eggs and then cooked them every way you can imagine; if any of the yolk remained liquid, the germs survived. If the eggs were then left at room temperature for any period of time, the bacteria grew rapidly.

Unpasteurized milk can be a greater risk than undercooked eggs. There are more varied disease-causing microbes in milk than eggs. Fortunately, pasteurization protects us against these microbes: in pasteurization, the milk is heated just hot enough to kill most (not all) bacteria but not hot enough to curdle the

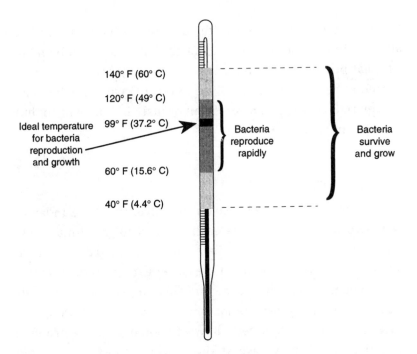

FIGURE 6.1 *The temperature danger zone for foods*
The temperature danger zone for food is 40°F to 140°F (4.4°C to 60°C).
Foods should be in the danger zone as little as possible and never for
more than one hour.

SOURCE: Adapted with permission from *Applied Food Service Sanitation*, 4th ed. (Washington,
D.C.: Educational Foundation of the National Restaurant Association, 1991): 132.

milk. When milk is not pasteurized, anyone who drinks it is
subject to get whatever bacteria are infecting the cow's udder.
For example, it is common for children who visit farms to taste
raw milk—and then get *Campylobacter* gastroenteritis. In Iowa,
one-third of the *Campylobacter* infections are associated with
raw milk ingestion.

Some rarer causes of food poisoning from animal products
are also worthy of mention. There are now fewer than fifty cases
of trichinosis a year in the United States. But when this parasitic infection of muscle occurs, it can be severe and life threatening. Undercooked pork and foods made of wild game, often

home-prepared sausages, are the usual culprits. Botulism has also become rare in the United States, but it, too, can be fatal. Of meat products, only homemade venison jerky has been reported to be a source of botulism in recent years. In table 6.2 I summarize how you can eat carnivorously if you want to, but not get infected.

Fish

May in Atlanta is high season for cookouts. One Sunday in May, two families in Atlanta each decided to grill tuna steak. The fish were bought from the same store, rinsed, seasoned, and grilled. Within fifteen minutes after eating, all diners were experiencing severe headache and flushing and were on their way to the emergency room. There, they were treated with Tylenol and antihistamines and were soon better. The problem was that the display case at the grocery store was not cool enough and the fish had spoiled. It did not look or smell bad, but it had formed sufficient toxin to make the people who ate it sick. What they had all experienced we call scombroid poisoning.

The symptoms of fish poisoning vary more than the symptoms of meat, dairy, or poultry poisoning. Although you will also get nausea, vomiting, and diarrhea after eating bad fish, a range of other more specific problems may occur. In scombroid poisoning, the bacteria that normally inhabit the fish, given enough time at a fitting temperature, degrade histidine in the meat to histamine. Histamine is the same substance that the human body's blood cells release to cause common allergic symptoms, so scombroid is a lot like a severe allergic attack. Scombroid poisoning is especially associated with dark-meated fish, particularly the large bony fish with oily flesh, like tuna and mackerel. A metallic, peppery taste is sometimes noted, but usually the fish looks, smells, and tastes normal. Only

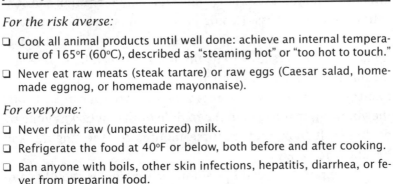

TABLE 6.2
Rules for preventing foodborne diseases from meat, dairy, poultry, and eggs

For the risk averse:

❑ Cook all animal products until well done: achieve an internal temperature of 165°F (60°C), described as "steaming hot" or "too hot to touch."

❑ Never eat raw meats (steak tartare) or raw eggs (Caesar salad, homemade eggnog, or homemade mayonnaise).

For everyone:

❑ Never drink raw (unpasteurized) milk.

❑ Refrigerate the food at 40°F or below, both before and after cooking.

❑ Ban anyone with boils, other skin infections, hepatitis, diarrhea, or fever from preparing food.

proper refrigeration, all along the way, will prevent scombroid poisoning. Cooking does not destroy the toxin.

The most common fish poisoning is ciguatera. This is also caused by a toxin that resists heat, so cooking the fish will not prevent the problem. This toxin, not surprisingly called ciguatoxin, is first made by microorganisms. The microorganisms that produce ciguatoxin are protozoans that live on or near tropical reefs. Even though they're the same kind of protozoans that cause red tides, there's usually no way to tell when a reef is contaminated. Small invertebrates ingest the protozoans and then the toxin passes right up the food chain without being destroyed. Ultimately, it becomes concentrated in the meat of large bottom feeders like grouper, red snapper, and amberjack. Barracuda so commonly causes ciguatera that it has been banned as a food in Miami. You are most likely to get ciguatera from a tropical dinner, but because the toxin also resists freezing, this problem can show up anywhere fresh frozen fish is served.

You've long completed an apparently normal meal before the symptoms of ciguatera fish poisoning begin. Five hours is the average incubation period. As with most food poisonings, the gastrointestinal tract is affected first. The nausea, vomiting, and diarrhea are over quickly. But then the nerves become affected and that lasts a long time. You may feel abnormal sensations and weakness. Itching is common; so are burning and stinging sensations on the arms and legs. Hot and cold sensations can be reversed. Rarely, the weakness can be severe and incapacitating. This can all be gone in a day or it can last months. After my own parents dined on grouper in St. Croix, the vomiting that began in the middle of the night was gone by daybreak. It took another three months for the tingling and tiredness to go away.

Eating raw fish (sushi, sashimi, or ceviche) is rapidly gaining popularity in the United States. There are several special problems that are associated with eating raw fish. For example, fish can carry various worms. Anisakiasis is a common infection humans can get after ingesting the worm parasites of fish. It can cause abrupt nausea and vomiting or be more chronic and mimic peptic ulcers or colitis. Some students became patients of mine because of a different parasite transmitted from raw fish. They had decided to make their own sushi. When they later discovered they were excreting parts of the fish tapeworm, they realized that preparing sushi and sashimi is the province of an expert.

If you enjoy eating raw fish, the way to avoid infection is to limit yourself to eating sushi at reputable establishments whose personnel have the proper expertise. In that case, the fish will be monitored closely and the food will be prepared by a trained chef who can recognize and discard infected parts. Fugu, the Japanese puffer fish, is an extreme example of why preparing raw fish requires expertise. Although fugu is considered a delicacy, the fugu chef must clean the fish in an exacting manner. (In Japan, the chef requires a license.) The viscera, which contain a toxin called tetrodotoxin, must be carefully separated from the flesh. Tetrodotoxin is usually deadly. (See table 6.3 for ways to avoid fish poisoning generally.)

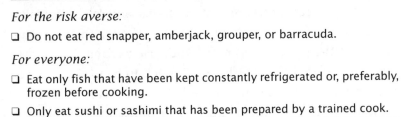

TABLE 6.3
Protecting yourself from tainted fish

For the risk averse:

❏ Do not eat red snapper, amberjack, grouper, or barracuda.

For everyone:

❏ Eat only fish that have been kept constantly refrigerated or, preferably, frozen before cooking.

❏ Only eat sushi or sashimi that has been prepared by a trained cook.

Botulism is a potentially deadly food poisoning. It could be included in any section of this chapter because any type of stored food contaminated by the spores of the bacterium *Clostridium botulinum* can cause it. But most recent reports of botulism have involved various ethnic groups' methods of using dried seafood. Cases have followed ingestion of ribytz, the salted air-dried whitefish of Russian immigrants; palani, the Hawaiian delicacy made from a reef scavenger; molahe, uneviscerated salt-dried fish favored by Egyptian-Americans; and whale meat stored in oil by Inuit people. In the past, botulism was most common after eating foods that had been canned at home without meticulous sterilizing. Botulism is a serious illness; it kills one-fifth of its victims. About a day after eating the tainted food, one experiences progressive weakness. It starts with dry mouth, blurred vision, and difficulty swallowing. The weakness then descends from the head to the rest of the body. Some botulism patients become too weak to breathe.

Any time food is left at room temperature for over sixteen hours before eating, the people who eat it are at risk for botulism. Sixteen hours is enough time for the bacteria to release sufficient toxin into the food. But cooking is an effective way to destroy this toxin. Boiling for ten minutes or heating to 80°F for thirty minutes works.

Shellfish

Many kinds of shellfish are filter feeders. The ones that present the biggest risk are oysters, clams, and mussels, which siphon relatively large volumes of water through their systems to extract the particles of matter they use as food. In the process, any viruses or bacteria that happen to be in the water or bottom mud become concentrated. An oyster can accumulate a concentration of viruses up to 100 times greater than the concentration in the water surrounding it. And still we prefer to eat shellfish whole and raw or briefly steamed. It is no wonder that a wide range of infections and intoxications (poisonings) have been transmitted from mollusks to people who eat them raw. Table 6.4 lists many of these, though it may be an incomplete list; in some outbreaks no specific etiology is found and epidemiologists suspect that shellfish carry viruses that we still cannot identify.

If this were a perfect world, raw shellfish would be safer. Oyster beds would always be protected from contamination by sewage and shellfish would reliably be cleansed after harvesting by depuration—that is, feeding them in purified water for three days. But rules get broken, and purging with clean water is not completely effective. In 1988, sixty-eight people in Florida developed viral hepatitis A from eating the same batch of raw oysters. The oysters had been harvested from outside the authorized zones and in an area where both a sewage plant and boats deposited effluent. This could easily happen again.

In addition, some pathogens that become concentrated in oysters and clams are not the result of contamination but are normal to the marine environment. Depuration does not rid shellfish of these. For example, *Vibrio vulnificus* is a bacterium that normally lives in coastal waters; it can cause a gastroenteritis that may be fatal, especially to those with liver disease. Another marine bacterium, *Vibrio parahemolyticus*, is also part of the ocean's normal microorganismal flora. It is the cause of

TABLE 6.4
Infections and intoxications from shellfish

Campylobacter	Shellfish poisoning
Cholera	Toxigenic *E. coli*
Hepatitis A	Typhoid fever
Norovirus	*Vibrio parahemolyticus*
Plesiomonas	*Vibrio vulnificus*

half the gastroenteritis in Japan, but is less common in North America. It causes a bloody diarrhea. You can get this pathogen from oysters, but more commonly from crabs, shrimp, and lobsters that have been inadequately cooked or refrigerated. Cholera is also a type of *Vibrio* infection. It is extremely rare in the United States but can be transmitted in inadequately cooked Gulf Coast crabs or oysters. (For more on cholera, see chapter 7.)

The most common infection after eating shellfish is caused by norovirus. This garden-variety gastroenteritis—nausea, vomiting, and diarrhea starting a day after eating raw clams or oysters—lasts one or two days. Norovirus may also be acquired from contaminated surfaces or infected food handlers. Adequate cooking will protect you from most infections transmitted by shellfish, including norovirus infection. If you are steaming the shellfish, fifteen minutes is necessary. (Steaming for only five minutes is not an uncommon practice.)

There is one instance in which cooking will not help to purify a shellfish, but it is quite rare. It is called shellfish poisoning and is caused by a toxin (called saxitoxin) that is undaunted by cooking. This toxin only occurs in cooler latitudes (above 30 degrees north) between May and October, especially after red tides. This type of shellfish poisoning causes numbness, tingling, muscular weakness, and other neurologic problems, starting only a few minutes after ingesting the tainted mussels, clams, oysters, or scallops. (Table 6.5 lists suggestions for avoiding illness associated with seafood.)

TABLE 6.5
Safer seafood

For the risk averse:

❏ Eat no raw shellfish.

For everyone:

❏ If you are steaming seafood, cook it for at least 15 minutes.

❏ Eat sushi and sashimi only if prepared by a trained cook.

❏ If you have heard that there is a red tide along a stretch of coastline, do not eat shellfish harvested from that area.

❏ If you will be eating raw oysters, get the hepatitis A vaccine, unless you've already had hepatitis A.

Vegetables

On a Sunday, March 31, 1993, 202 people enjoyed an apparently healthy buffet dinner at a lodge in New Hampshire. The remainder of the weekend was eventful. An average of thirty-eight hours later, over three-quarters of the diners developed profuse watery diarrhea with cramps. What everyone in this group had in common was consumption of the same tabouleh salad, made with vegetables grown in the United States and prepared early the night before. These people were all infected with a toxin-producing bacterium, *E. coli*. The strains of *E. coli* found on vegetables are usually different from the kind common on hamburgers. The *E. coli* on vegetables cause bad gastroenteritis that starts about a day after eating a contaminated salad; the infection can last for up to a week.

E. coli is not the only offender when it comes to food poisoning from vegetables. *Shigella*, *Listeria*, and *Clostridium* can cause it, too. The good thing about vegetables, though, is that the contamination is just on their surface. The offending germs can be washed off before the vegetables are prepared for eating. Proper refrigeration is still critical.

Often, the food poisoning associated with salads has nothing to do with the vegetables, but with the salad dressing and seasonings—and the cook. Salads made with mayonnaise are infamous for causing staphylococcal poisoning, the most common type of food poisoning of all. *Staphylococcus aureus* ("staph" for short) is the bacterium responsible for common skin infections, like boils. But it also produces various toxins. (Toxic shock syndrome is usually the result of one of staph's toxins.) If staph have been given time to grow in a salad and release a toxin, you can't tell that when you sit down to eat. But you'll know within just a few hours when the profuse vomiting starts. Staphylococcal food poisoning is quite unpleasant, but it doesn't cause much diarrhea and lasts no longer than a day.

It takes three things to set the stage for staphylococcal food poisoning: a cook carrying *Staphylococcus aureus* who gets it on the food, a food on which staph likes to grow, and a period of time in warm conditions for the bacteria to multiply. Foods with plenty of salt and/or sugar are havens for staph. Macaroni salad, potato salad, and the like are perfect, and ham, custard, pastries, and many other foods have all been associated with staphylococcal food poisoning from time to time.

If you are eating out, the only thing I can advise is to avoid the salad altogether if you do not believe a salad has been continuously cooled. When preparing vegetables yourself, wash them thoroughly with a diluted, mild detergent, and rinse that off completely with subsequent rinses of clean water. Use clean utensils and cutting boards. Except when actually doing the preparing, keep the vegetables and dressing in the refrigerator.

Anyone with any sort of skin infection (impetigo, boils, or folliculitis) or with uncontrolled eczema should stay out of the kitchen. And cooks must keep their fingers out of their nose! If a person carries *Staphylococcus aureus* on their body, it concentrates in their nose; a cook must be careful not to transfer

TABLE 6.6
Secure salads

___

❑ Wash all vegetables in a dilute, mild detergent and then rinse copiously.

❑ Except when actually preparing salads, keep salads refrigerated, just like all other foods.

❑ Exclude from the kitchen anyone with a known or suspected staph infection, gastroenteritis, or diarrhea.

___

staph from that reservoir to the food being prepared. (See table 6.6 for ways to keep salads safe to eat.)

Water

In April 1993, the people of Milwaukee found out that our tap water is not always germ-free: more than 400,000 persons there came down with an infection called cryptosporidiosis, transmitted in the city's tap water. This infection is caused by *Cryptosporidium parvum,* a one-celled parasite whose cysts can live quite happily in ordinary drinking water. (One of Milwaukee's water treatment plants was contaminated with these cysts, but how that occurred isn't known.) The diarrhea of cryptosporidiosis may last for a month in people with intact immune systems, but may not get better on its own in people with HIV infection.

The Milwaukee outbreak was the largest of its kind on record, but there have been many smaller outbreaks of this parasite or other pathogens that find their way into drinking water. Although tap water in the United States is almost always safe, it isn't usually checked for the microscopic cysts of *Cryptosporidium,* and *Cryptosporidium* is not affected by chlorination. Some household tap water filters that are currently on the market do not strain out these organisms either. People who are very susceptible to enteric illness (that is, those with HIV or those who have had an organ transplant) might want to eat and drink as if they were traveling in a country where the risk of contaminated food and water is high (see table 7.1). All of us should be suspicious if we see turbid water come from the tap—there might be a breach in the water treatment system.

Cryptosporidium parvum can also find its way into swimming pools, usually from an infected child who is excreting the cysts. Since an infected person excretes very large numbers of cysts and the parasite is immune to chlorine, swimming pools are another place cryptosporidiosis is spread. Large outbreaks have occurred at amusement park "wave pools," where splashing favors ingestion of water.

When you are in the country or camping, you really have to watch what you drink. Well water or surface water must never be taken downhill from a septic tank or any other area of waste disposal. Surface water may be contaminated, in any case, by the germs excreted from animals living upstream. These germs include *Cryptosporidium, Campylobacter*, and *Salmonella*, but *Giardia* is by far the most prevalent. This parasite lives in the intestines of beaver, muskrat, goats, sheep, cattle, and mule deer. Ingesting as few as ten microscopic *Giardia* cysts can start this infection. (The cysts resist stomach acid.)

If you go camping for a weekend and drink contaminated surface water, you probably won't become ill while you're out there; giardiasis has an incubation period that can usually be measured in weeks. But when it starts, it can be terribly unpleasant. The diarrhea is associated with much gas (belching, bloating, and flatulence), and without treatment it can last for months or even years, its symptoms waxing and waning. The best preventive approach is to purify all surface water before using it.

The two best means of purifying surface water for drinking are boiling and adding iodine. Keeping water at a rolling boil for one minute is sufficient. The tincture of iodine (2 percent) sold for treating cuts is the same used for purifying water. Add five drops per quart of water, twice that if the water is cloudy. Letting the treated water stand for thirty minutes will eliminate bacteria, but to effectively eliminate *Giardia* cysts you must allow the water to sit overnight (eight hours). Some commercial iodine products (for example, Potable Aqua) will do the same thing, but chlorine-based products (bleach or Halazone) are less effective. Outdoor stores also sell filtration systems for hikers to use to rid their drinking water of *Giardia* cysts. Dr. Jerry Ongerth and others at the University of Washington tested these and found only two of them to really work: First Need Water Purification Device and Katadyn Pocket Filter. Some of the other filters they tested let through almost all of the cysts!

Pets

The infections we get from our pets are not, strictly speaking, food poisoning. But we often get so close to our pets that whatever germs they carry are likely to get onto our hands—and then get into our mouths. The animals we cherish often carry bacteria that cause gastroenteritis. Animals, of course, get a wide range of infections, but most of these infections cannot be transmitted to people. We are at risk, though, for several of our pets' germs. People often get diarrhea from *Campylobacter* bacteria transmitted from dogs, cats, birds, goats, hamsters, sheep, and turtles; a puppy with diarrhea is perhaps the most common source. The bacteria *Salmonella* on amphibians and reptiles can also cause human diarrhea; when turtles were common household pets, exposure to them accounted for 14 percent of all cases of salmonellosis in the United States. Snakes and lizards commonly carry *Salmonella*, but dogs, cats, and birds can, too.

You cannot always tell if your pet is a carrier of one of these bacteria because the pet may not necessarily become ill. Whenever a pet does have loose stools, be especially careful. Keep children away; they have the closest contact with our pets during play. Wash your hands after contact with a sick pet and use bleach to wash down the animal's cage, house, pen, and waste box. Bleach is a good disinfectant: it will work best if you let it sit on surfaces for fifteen minutes before you wipe it off. By all means, get your pet to the veterinarian.

Even if you are aware that your pet has, say, *Salmonella*, the veterinarian may not be able to do anything about it. It is not uncommon for healthy pets (or people) to carry *Salmonella* for long periods of time, even if they've received antibiotics. Even if your pets seem healthy, clean and disinfect pets' living spaces from time to time. Prevent pets from excreting feces in kids' sandboxes. If you keep amphibians or reptiles as pets, take special care to follow all these rules.

We do not live in a sterile environment. That's okay the vast majority of the time: our bodies are well equipped to keep out harmful microorganisms and toxins. When it comes to what you eat and drink, though, you want to be particularly careful. In this chapter, I have tried to give you a plan for doing just that.

7   *Health hazards of travel*

*T*ravel is marvelous. Illness is dreadful. All too often, the two go together. With only a bit of care, though, the pleasure of travel can remain unspoiled by the pain of sickness.

To avoid illness, some kinds of trips require almost no preparation. A business trip to a major capital, for example, is generally quite safe and easy to get ready for. Most of the time you'll be at risk for little else than traveler's diarrhea. On the other hand, sometimes advanced planning can literally be lifesaving. A hunting or birding trip in the tropics is fraught with hazards, although all of them are avoidable. You really can go anywhere on the globe and do almost anything imaginable and remain free of infection—if you plan properly and follow some simple rules.

The infections you can encounter abroad are literally innumerable, but many of them generally affect only the local population. Travelers actually acquire relatively few kinds of infections, so it is easy to focus on preventive strategies for the most common afflictions. These infections are best categorized by the ways they are spread: infections carried by food and water, those transmitted by the bites of insects, airborne infections, and those that pass through the skin.

Shots and drugs can be important, but avoiding the initial contact with the offending germs is even more important. For instance, in 1992, on its way to LA, Argentinas Flight number 386 made a stop in Lima, Peru. The food and/or water they picked up there was contaminated with cholera bacteria and

TABLE 7.1
Cardinal rules for eating abroad

Do:

❑ Eat only foods that have recently been fully cooked or freshly peeled

❑ Drink local beverages only if they are carbonated or have been recently boiled

Don't:

❑ Eat salads

❑ Eat garnishes

❑ Add unboiled milk or cream

❑ Drink locally bottled water

❑ Drink water on an airplane leaving an airport abroad

❑ Add ice or suck on ice

❑ Eat food from street vendors

❑ Brush teeth with tap water

NOTE: These rules apply everywhere outside the United States, Canada, Western Europe, Japan, Australia, and New Zealand.

---

85 of the 356 people aboard contracted cholera. One died. Had they all been immunized, most still would have become ill, but had they all followed the cardinal rules for eating abroad (table 7.1), few would have. The most common infection from insects, malaria, is now often resistant to drugs, but if you avoid insect bites you avoid malaria. Two college students became paraplegic in 1984 from a worm infection called schistosomiasis. They became infected by swimming in a river in Kenya. They each had had all the appropriate shots and pills; there is no vaccine for this infection. Again, avoidance is key.

In the following four sections, I will tell you about the major diseases for which travelers are at risk. I will group them by the four modes by which they are spread. The strategy for avoiding the entire group of diseases will be highlighted first. Then, specific prevention strategies will be detailed for each specific disease. Finally, I will outline how to make an overall plan for a given trip and give suggestions about where to get the best help, both home and abroad.

Infections from food and water

Most travelers' infections are contracted by ingestion. Diarrhea is the most common disorder to affect visitors to developing counties. (It is also the most frequent illness associated with war in these regions and so has been an area of careful research done by the military.) But simple diarrhea is only one of many diseases contracted by travelers from food and water. Other enteric illnesses include cholera, typhoid fever, amebic dysentery, polio, brucellosis, hepatitis A, and a wide array of intestinal parasites, including tapeworms and *Giardia*. One set of rules will prevent this entire class of enteric illnesses.

You must be sure that food and drink are not contaminated. Heat, carbonation, and alcohol are the most convenient tools to use to ensure that. (Filters by themselves are not reliable; use one of these other methods for insurance.)

Heat kills germs. Food should reach 160°F (71°C) throughout to kill bacteria. So if you are served food that is steaming hot (too hot to eat without cooling first), you can feel confident that it is sterile. Consider sending a meal back if you don't think it has been fully cooked. Boiled fluids like coffee and tea are also safe. The heat of baking will sterilize breads, and they will stay safe indefinitely because they are dry. Pasteurization is also a heat sterilization process. If you buy milk or butter in a closed container clearly marked "pasteurized," from an apparently reliable company, it is also fit for consumption.

Carbonation will also render your beverages safe to drink. The bubbles in carbonated beverages are carbon dioxide. Some of that CO_2 is forming carbonic acid at all times. Given time, carbonic acid is lethal to the bacteria, viruses, and parasites that cause enteric illness. Learn the phrases *con gas, avec gazeuse,* or the appropriate equivalents before your trip.

Alcohol is likewise a germicide, but, like carbonation, it does not work instantaneously. Therefore, wine and beer are fine, but a mixed drink is only as sterile as the mixer and the ice. Ice can actually be a germ preservative, and more than one traveler has unknowingly ordered "dysentery on the rocks."

A wise precaution is to buy a few small plastic bottles of water or seltzer before leaving home and keep one with you. Then you'll have clean water on hand to swig when you hit a chili pepper in a local dish or when you are brushing your teeth in the hotel room. A more lightweight solution is to bring along tincture of iodine. Five drops of the standard tincture of iodine (2 percent), available at most pharmacies, will effectively sterilize a quart of clear water of bacteria (and hepatitis A). Use ten drops per quart if the water is cloudy. Remember that iodine takes thirty minutes to work. Whenever you are traveling, think twice about anything that goes into your mouth. If a lake is contaminated, even the small amounts of water consumed when swimming can make you very sick!

Whereas iodine treatment will effectively kill bacteria— and bacteria are by far the most common intestinal threat to travelers—only boiling will reliably eliminate protozoan cysts from drinking water. Although less common, these parasites (*Giardia, Cryptosporidium,* and *Cyclospora*) can each cause protracted intestinal infections, and each is widely distributed in the drinking water of developing countries. The careful traveler who wants to avoid these protozoa will stick to boiling as a means of sterilizing local water. Maintaining a rolling boil for one minute is sufficient.

Traveler's diarrhea. Have you heard this old wisecrack: "Travel broadens the mind and loosens the bowels"? Diarrhea is a common, everyday affair in the developing world. Locals do get partially immune, but, as Dr. Herb DuPont (a tall Texan whose self-described research focus has been "crap") puts it, "travelers are immunologically like children." Your risk of developing traveler's diarrhea during short-term travel to, say, Mexico, is 20 to 50 percent. If you stay, there is a 90 percent chance you will experience diarrhea by month nine. If you visit a developing nation and you are young, have an adventurous travel style, or have your protective stomach acid neutralized (by an antacid), you are even more likely to get traveler's diarrhea, and get it sooner. Travel to an industrialized nation does not pose nearly so high a risk.

When you do develop traveler's diarrhea, here's what you can expect: on average, a total of four to five loose stools during a four- to five-day period. The odds are two in three that you'll have cramps as well. You are less likely to experience nausea, vomiting (a 10 percent chance), or fever (also 10 percent). Traveler's diarrhea can be caused by viruses, parasites, or bacteria ingested in food or water, but usually it is from bacteria called enterotoxigenic *Escherichia coli* ingested with food.

If you truly pay heed to the cardinal rules for eating abroad, you have a very good chance of escaping traveler's diarrhea. But, just in case, be prepared with the right remedies. The military and Dr. DuPont have shown that proper treatment can shorten the length of illness to only one hour. To accomplish this, you must start treatment at the first suspicious whiff or gush. You must have with you and take two different medicines: an antidiarrhea medicine that slows bowel contractions and an antibiotic to kill the infecting germs.

The safest medicine of the antidiarrhea variety is Imodium. It comes in 2-milligram (mg) capsules without a prescription. Take two after the first loose bowel movement and then one after each subsequent episode. Do not give Imodium to young children.

Currently, the best antibiotics for traveler's diarrhea are called quinolones; for example, gatifloxacin (Tequin) 400 mg, ciprofloxacin (Cipro) 500 mg, and norfloxacin (Noroxin) 400 mg. Take for three days. Have compassion and carry enough for a travel mate. In the United States, you will need a prescription for these quinolones. In most other countries, you can probably pick these medicines up in a pharmacy without a prescription. Do not take a quinolone if you are under eighteen, pregnant, or allergic to this kind of antibiotic. If you are younger than eighteen and not allergic to sulfa drugs, substitute sulfamethoxazole-trimethoprim (Septra, Bactrim). This agent is currently less reliable than quinolones. For example, only half the strains of *Escherichia coli* isolated in Saudi Arabia and Kuwait are susceptible to Septra, but in the interior of Mexico it still works. Do not take Septra if you might be pregnant or are allergic to sulfa drugs.

If your traveler's diarrhea is worse than I have described—if you have high fever or bloody stools—seek reliable medical advice instead of self-treatment. In that case, if there is any delay in seeing the doctor, it is important not to slow the bowels (don't take the Imodium), but it is imperative to stay hydrated. Drink, drink, drink! If you can, replace the volume of lost fluid approximately ounce for ounce. Besides fluid replacement, replacing your electrolytes (minerals dissolved in blood) is important, too. So, choose a fluid to drink that is designed to accomplish that. The oral rehydration solution promoted by the World Health Organization is available commercially and will do this, as will other brands, such as Pedialyte and Stop Trot. The simplest oral rehydration solution to make yourself is one level teaspoon of table salt plus four heaping teaspoons of sugar added to one liter of potable water.

Some advocate taking prophylactic antibiotics for traveler's diarrhea. I do not. Here's why: Taking medicines is a bother under any circumstances, and more so while traveling. If you follow the rules, the odds are against your becoming ill, yet the antibiotics themselves can cause side effects. (There is about a 3 percent risk.) Furthermore, a preventive medicine may give you a false sense of security. If you go ahead and break the dietary rules, you are likely to get infected with a germ resistant to whatever you were taking.

If you feel you absolutely must take some kind of preventive medicine, then bismuth subsalicylate (Pepto-Bismol) is best. Two tablets with meals and two again at bedtime (a total of eight) can reduce risk of traveler's diarrhea by two-thirds, and you are not using up an antibiotic option that may be needed later. This regimen will turn your stools black and might do the same to your tongue. Note: if you shouldn't take aspirin, you should not take Pepto-Bismol.

Polio. North Americans think of polio as a disease that has been vanquished, but in parts of Asia, the Indian subcontinent, and sub-Saharan Africa, new cases still may occur. Polio is caused by a virus spread through contaminated water. If you follow the cardinal rules about avoiding contaminated water, you should not catch polio. However, the disease is so devastating and immunization is so effective that you should ensure your status before travel to any destination where transmission of polio is still occurring.

If you have never received polio vaccine, you will need a primary series of three doses. But most travelers will need only a single booster. We no longer recommend the oral polio vaccine, the one you may have been given to swallow as a child. This is because some individuals (especially those over eighteen years old who have never before taken the oral polio vaccine, and persons with an immune deficiency) have a risk of catching polio from the vaccine itself. That's because the vaccine contains live virus. We now give only an injectable vaccine called the enhanced inactivated polio vaccine. This vaccine is made up of killed virus and cannot give you polio.

Hepatitis A. Hepatitis A is another virus that you ingest and that is a common risk overseas. I will cover it in more detail in chapter 11. It is worthwhile getting a shot to prevent hepatitis A before you travel to the developing world. For many years, the shot given was gamma globulin, a 2-cc injection to protect you for four months and a 5-cc dose for five to twelve months. Gamma globulin is safe and effective for this purpose. However, a new hepatitis A vaccine is now available. It is also quite safe and has some advantages over the globulin. The vaccine can offer more long-lived protection from hepatitis A virus, has fewer interactions with other shots you might also need before your trip, and, unlike the globulin, is not made from a human blood product. Take hepatitis A vaccine two weeks or more before you depart so that it will have time to work before you need it.

Cholera. Cholera occurs in worldwide epidemics called pandemics. Six of these occurred before the twentieth century, but the seventh cholera pandemic began in 1961 and is ongoing. Although it started and continues in Asia, in 1991 cholera struck Peru. By 1992, over 45,000 cases and 4,000 deaths occurred there. The disease is now spreading and reaching north into Mexico, east through Brazil, and south into Argentina. Although it is very unlikely that you would contract cholera in the United States, a case a week now occurs here in persons returning from countries in Latin America, Asia, and Africa.

Cholera is caused by a bacterium (*Vibrio cholera*). The toxin released by this germ produces watery diarrhea that is so profuse that one goes into shock if the fluids and electrolytes are not promptly replaced. *Vibrio cholera* is particularly found on shellfish—it adheres to the chitin of their shells. (A good example of a meal likely to put you in jeopardy for cholera would be a fresh seafood salad in Ecuador or Cambodia, sites of two recently reported epidemics.) Again, the key to avoiding cholera is not ingesting the germs; be sure any viable organisms in food or water have been rendered inactive by heat, carbonation, alcohol, or iodine, as advised earlier.

There is a cholera vaccine, but it is not very effective protection against most strains of the bacteria, and it does not protect you at all from the newest epidemic strain (strain 0139). Moreover, it can cause severe local reactions, if not a flulike illness. I do not recommend the cholera vaccine. There are no cholera vaccine requirements for entry or exit in any Latin American country or the United States. No country will ask for proof of cholera vaccine when you are arriving from the United States. Occasionally, though, local officials may want to see cholera vaccination certificates if you are arriving from certain other countries. Call the appropriate embassy to check whether you'll be required to have the vaccination. If you find that you will, ask your doctor ahead of time for a letter saying you cannot receive the vaccine. If absolutely necessary, get a single 0.5-cc injection. This will satisfy the officials.

Typhoid. Typhoid fever is one more disease caused by a bacterium (*Salmonella typhi*) you can ingest in contaminated food or drink. Typhoid causes high fevers and the invasion of the bloodstream by bacteria, and it may be fatal. Risk to travelers is generally quite low, but may be up to twenty times higher in certain areas, including India and Peru.

Although never officially required, two new vaccines have become available. An oral vaccine called *Salmonella typhi* Ty21a was released in 1989, and a new injectable typhoid vaccine, Typhim Vi, in 1995. Consider taking one or the other of them if you plan to travel off the usual tourist routes, whether or not you've ever received a typhoid vaccine previously. Each new vaccine is more effective and better tolerated than the century-old typhoid shots.

Salmonella typhi Ty21a can reduce your risk of contracting typhoid fever by 70 percent. It is taken in a series of pills. Each pill contains one billion bacteria that have been rendered harmless. That is, the bacteria can no longer cause the disease, but they can trigger your immune system to defend you against the harmful typhoid bacteria. You must take care to follow your doctor's and pharmacist's directions about handling this medication properly. The pills must be refrigerated (but not frozen) until use. Start the series at least two weeks before departure. Take a total of four pills, one pill every other day, one hour after meals. The immunity lasts for five years. This oral typhoid vaccine doesn't usually cause any side effects; occasionally it can cause nausea, vomiting, and headache. Like other live vaccines, Ty21a is not recommended for use in immune-deficient persons.

Typhim Vi must be given by injection, but it has the advantage of only requiring a single dose. If you choose to receive this variety of typhoid vaccine, you will have a 7 percent chance of developing a hard, red, tender reaction at the injection site. Typhim Vi is just about as effective as the oral Ty21a and will confer immunity for about two years.

Diseases from insect bites

Malaria is the most common serious health threat transmitted by insect bite, but there are literally hundreds of other diseases known to be spread by biting insects. These include yellow fever, elephantiasis, leishmaniasis (tropical sore), African sleeping sickness, dengue (or "breakbone") fever, and encephalitis. The insects that carry the organisms that cause these diseases are most likely to live in warm moist habitats, usually in the tropics or subtropics. (Ticks, which often live in temperate zones, strictly speaking, are not insects. See chapter 5 for information about tickborne diseases.)

The primary strategy for avoiding the whole lot of these diseases is obvious: avoid insect bites. How easily you can accomplish this depends on what activities you plan during your trip. Here are some basic rules to follow:

❑ Know when and where the disease-transmitting insects are most likely to be a problem. For example, the female *Anopheles* mosquito, which is the vector for malaria, feeds between dusk and dawn, generally in rural areas. But the *Aedes* mosquito, which transmits yellow fever and dengue fever, prefers to feed on humans during the daytime near towns.

❑ Whenever possible, keep your skin and head covered. Loose-fitting clothes are most effective at preventing insect bites.

❑ Try to spend as much time as you can in well-screened or air-conditioned areas. Mosquito netting over your bed at night may be useful.

❑ To get the best results from insect repellents, pick a repellent with DEET (*N,N*-diethyl-3-methylbenzamide) as its active ingredient. The optimal concentration of DEET is probably about 30 percent. Repellent may need to be reapplied if you get wet. Keep DEET away from eyes, nose, mouth, and open wounds, and be particularly careful using it on children.

❑ Spray a repellent that has permethrin (or pyrethrins) as the active ingredient on your clothes, on the walls of sleeping areas, and at flying insects. (Permanone is one brand.) This should stay effective for over a week if properly applied.

Malaria. Travel to the tropics is growing in popularity. As a parallel trend, the number of cases of malaria in Americans has increased. Over one thousand cases are brought back to the United States (and several times that to Europe) by travelers each year. People who emigrated from malarial regions (especially West Africa and India) to the United States often believe that they can visit their original countries without risk, that they are immune to malaria. They are wrong.

Malaria occurs widely throughout the tropics (see figure 7.1). You are at particularly high risk of infection in Papua New Guinea, the Solomon Islands, and sub-Saharan Africa. In all malarial regions, malaria is distributed in a spotty fashion. In Kenya, for example, (as surveyed in 1990 by Dr. Hans O. Lobel of the Centers of Disease Control) the highest risk is around Lake Victoria; it is intermediate on the coast, and lowest in the game parks (but still significant). These regional differences are nice to know, but I implore you to maintain effective precautions anyplace where malaria is endemic.

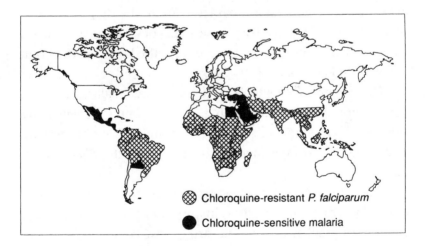

FIGURE 7.1 *Malaria in the world*

Source: Adapted from Centers for Disease Control, *Health Information for International Travel 1993* (Atlanta, Ga.: U.S. Department of Health and Human Services, 1993): 105.

TABLE 7.2
Symptoms of malaria

Common symptoms	Serious symptoms	Less common symptoms also seen
Fever	Mental confusion	Diarrhea
Chills	Lethargy	Abdominal pain
Sweats	Shortness of breath	Cough
Headache	Dark or bloody urine	Easy bleeding
Body aches		

Malaria is caused by a parasite known as *Plasmodium*, which is transmitted by the female *Anopheles* mosquito. We usually think of parasites living in the intestines or on the skin, but this one grows in red blood cells. After it matures in one set of blood cells, it ruptures them and seeks out a set of neighboring cells to live in and ultimately destroy. (It's a parasitic PacMan, as travel writer and malaria patient Tim Cahill puts it.) As the red blood cells rupture, infected persons experience hard shaking chills, fever, and sweats. Most patients have severe headaches. Later, when malaria parasites multiply, they clog small blood vessels. This can lead to serious complications or death when proper blood flow to the kidneys, the lungs, or the brain is hampered (see table 7.2).

There is no vaccine to protect you against malaria. Because you cannot be sure that clothing, mosquito nets, screens, and repellents will stop the *Anopheles* mosquito from biting you, you should also take medication that kills the *Plasmodium* parasites.

The medication that is best for you depends on your itinerary and your personal medical history. Since World War II, chloroquine (Aralen) has been the drug most commonly used to prevent malaria. Unfortunately, in many parts of the world, a strain of the malaria parasite, called chloroquine-resistant *Plasmodium falciparum* (CRPF), has become resistant to the medication. Those regions are clearly marked on the map, figure 7.1. Where the parasite is still sensitive to chloroquine, you need only take the medication. But in countries where CRPF is endemic, you should take another kind of preventive drug, mefloquine (Lariam).

You need to start taking these malaria pills before you ever arrive in the tropics so that medication is circulating (and you can spot side effects) before the first mosquito's buzz is heard. Each kind of medication is taken once weekly. Pick a day in the week that is convenient and easy to remember; many people choose Sunday. After you leave the malarial zone, you need to keep taking the medication for another four weeks (four doses) to kill any parasites just starting to develop in your body.

The medication you and your physician choose may depend on your personal medical history. See table 7.3 for a list of pre-cautions for each drug. Almost everyone can take chloroquine. If, however, you are entering an area with resistant malaria and cannot take mefloquine, consider taking doxycycline (Vibra-mycin). Unlike the other antimalarial drugs, doxycycline must be taken daily. Malarone is a new alternative. Note that chloro-quine may be acceptable in pregnancy, but the medications to prevent resistant malaria are not. Because malaria can be par-ticularly severe in pregnant women and because pregnant women should not take mefloquine or doxycycline, I urge preg-nant women to avoid travel to any malaria zone.

After you return from the tropics, as stated earlier, you still have to worry about malaria. You have to take your final month's worth of preventive medicine. Also, if you spent a month or more in a malaria zone, ask a knowledgeable physician about primaquine. This medication is sometimes needed to prevent malaria from relapsing; certain forms of malaria (specifically, *Plasmodium vivax* and *ovale*) can persist in your liver and reappear in your red blood cells even years after initial exposure. Finally, you need to keep a wary eye out for malaria symptoms.

TABLE 7.3
Drugs used to prevent malaria: precautions

Chloroquine (Aralen): Rarely this will cause nausea. It is better tolerated with meals and doses can be split, if necessary, so that half a dose is taken twice weekly.

Mefloquine (Lariam): If you have experienced seizures or if you are pregnant, do not take mefloquine. Mefloquine has a risk of exacerbating mental disorders.

Doxycycline (Vibramycin): This is not to be taken by anyone nine years old or younger, or by women who might be or become pregnant while taking it. It can cause nausea. It must be washed down well with food and/or drink or it will cause an ulcer.

Malarone: Must be taken daily. Expensive. Not safe in pregnancy.

That is because no manner of precaution is foolproof. Should you develop the symptoms of malaria (see table 7.2) anytime from one week to four *years* after being at risk, get checked for malaria. Many patients I have treated for malaria were first told they had "the flu" or given some other wrong diagnosis. The evaluation of fever, especially fever with headache, after visiting the tropics should include blood smears for malaria parasites.

Yellow fever. Yellow fever is another good reason to avoid mosquito bites in the tropics. Yellow fever causes a severe, often fatal form of hepatitis, locally sometimes called "the black vomit." The geographic range for yellow fever is more limited than for malaria (see figure 7.2). The disease is found in a band through equatorial Africa and South America. It is easier to prevent than malaria because there's a safe and highly effective vaccine for yellow fever. There are two good reasons to take this vaccine: it may be required by officials, and yellow fever is a disease with no known treatment.

Yellow fever vaccine is the only vaccine that other coun-

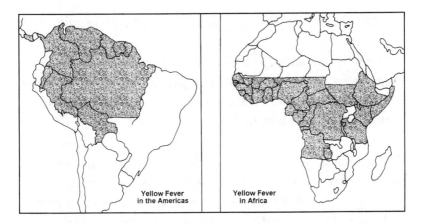

Yellow Fever
in the Americas

Yellow Fever
in Africa

FIGURE 7.2 *Yellow fever in the world*
Source: Adapted from Centers for Disease Control, *Health Information for International Travel 1993* (Atlanta, Ga.: U.S. Department of Health and Human Services, 1993): 137–138.

tries might require travelers from the United States to show proof of. Call your local health department or travel clinic to find out where and when they give it. The vaccine is only given at Public Health Service clinics or their licensees, and one vial of vaccine is good for only one hour after it is activated; therefore, yellow fever vaccine is generally given only once a week at a specified clinic and time.

There are only two groups of people who should not get this vaccine: those with egg allergy and those with poor immune function. The vaccine is made in chicken eggs; if you are allergic to eggs, you should not have the yellow fever vaccine. Because vaccine is made from live virus, anyone whose immune system has difficulty controlling viruses (such as patients with HIV infection or lymphoma) should not take it. A vaccination for yellow fever stays effective for ten years.

Japanese B encephalitis. Many people who are infected with Japanese B encephalitis don't even become ill. However, if you do get sick from this virus, you'll have a 30 percent chance of dying and another 30 percent chance of having permanent brain damage. There is no good treatment. Again, prevention is so important.

Despite its name, this virus infection is more common in other Asian countries than it is in Japan. It is found throughout Asia. Although it is one of many viral diseases that are carried by mosquitos and that infect the brain, I single this one out because a vaccine is available. Most travelers don't need the vaccine because their risk is so low and allergic reactions to the vaccine can be severe. Nevertheless, if you will be traveling to Asia, staying for a prolonged visit—two weeks or more—and spending a significant amount of time in rural areas, consider taking this immunization.

The vaccine is given in a series of two or three doses given one or two weeks apart and has limited availability. You'll have to request information from the CDC, a travel clinic, and/or embassies to learn whether there is indeed risk at your destination(s) during the months you'll be there and to find out where you can be immunized.

Infections that spread through the air

Infections caused by pathogens that you breathe in with the air are not unique to the developing world or to travelers. Indeed, such airborne infections happen in the United States, only at a much lower rate. When you travel to countries whose public health systems are limited, however, you encounter airborne diseases that used to be common worldwide. These include measles, tuberculosis, meningitis, diphtheria, and influenza.

Most diseases in this class get spread by the coughs, breaths, and sneezes of infected people in crowded places with poor ventilation. Try to avoid crowds in enclosed buildings or vehicles when you travel in places where the general health of the populace is not optimal. A long ride on a public bus is an example of this kind of risk. So is a long airplane trip. The biggest worry in such settings is tuberculosis. Tuberculosis (TB) warrants its own chapter (see chapter 9), but it is worth repeating that Africa and Asia have particularly high levels of TB.

Measles. Measles (medically termed rubeola) has not been eradicated, even in the United States. This is a matter of consternation for the public health community because effective vaccination is widely available. In the United States, the disease is now limited to occasional outbreaks, but many more cases occur in other countries where fewer persons are vaccinated.

Measles is caused by an airborne virus. You breathe in the virus when you are close to an infected person. Cough, red watery eyes, fever, and a skin rash are the usual signs of measles. The most worrisome aspect of measles is an associated pneumonia that happens only in the very young, the very old, and in others whose immune system is not up to speed.

You only get measles once. If you know you've had them, don't worry. Also, if you were born before 1957, before kids began to be immunized against measles, you can assume you have had measles because almost all children did back then. There have been some problems with older vaccines, so only assume you have been rendered immune by vaccination if your records show you have received it since 1980. If you don't qualify as immune to measles, you should receive measles vaccine before you travel abroad. All children should now receive a measles vaccine booster at age twelve. (Colleges usually require proof of a measles booster before admission.)

It is usual and advisable to get vaccinated for mumps and rubella (German measles) right along with measles. The vaccine comes as a three-in-one injection and is called MMR. If you are already immune to any of the three, it won't hurt to get the additional dose. But since rubella vaccine can theoretically pose a risk to a fetus, women will want to receive MMR only when they are sure they are not pregnant—during menses, for example. Some immune-deficient persons should also forgo measles vaccine or MMR because these are live virus vaccines.

Meningitis. The most menacing type of meningitis, that caused by *Meningococcus* bacteria, can be a risk for travelers. Although these meningitis bacteria infect your nervous system, they get there through your lungs or nasal passages. A safe, effective vaccine is available that can prevent the bacteria from invading your airways. Travelers who may spend time among crowds of people in countries in which meningitis has been epidemic or in areas where meningitis is always prevalent (Saudi Arabia and sub-Saharan Africa) should get vaccinated before they leave the United States. Proof of vaccination is required to attend the Hajj. This meningitis vaccine, called quadrivalent meningococcal vaccine, offers protection against four of the most common strains of *Meningococcus*, but at least nine other strains exist. So, it is still best to cover your mouth and nose in crowds if you feel you might get coughed on.

Influenza. Influenza (flu) viruses are named after Asian places because they start there. Flu spreads from west to east yearly. In the United States, it is best to get the influenza vaccine in early November, but travelers should consider getting it earlier in the year (see chapter 8). One version of flu vaccine is available all year.

Diphtheria. Diphtheria is basically a terrible sore throat. It is caused by the bacterium *Corynebacterium diphtheriae.* This bacterium can form a membrane that may block your airway and/or release a toxin that can cause a kind of nerve poisoning. Whenever immunization levels wane in a population, diphtheria cases surge. In the former Soviet Union, many new cases occurred in the 1990s: over seven hundred cases and twenty-four deaths were recognized in Moscow alone in 1992. The diphtheria vaccine is quite safe and is given to adults as a "Td" shot, in combination with tetanus toxoid. Get a booster of Td if ten or more years have elapsed since your last one.

Infections contracted through the skin

You can get some infections from animal bites and some through wounds, but you can also contract disease through normal, intact skin. The general guidelines here are straightforward. Clean and cover any break in the skin, be it a minor abrasion or deeper laceration. Use soap and copious sterile water first, a germicide (for example, Betadine) from your kit (table 7.4) next, and then bandage the wound.

Tetanus. Tetanus is a life-threatening disease that can be caused by even trivial wounds. If a wound becomes contami-

---

TABLE 7.4
Contents of an infection protection travel kit

Bottled water
For diarrhea:
    Imodium
    An antibiotic (see text)
For wounds:
    A germicide such as Betadine or Neosporin
    Band-Aids
    An antibiotic such as dicloxacillin
Iodine or filter for water purification
Acetaminophen (Tylenol) for fever or pain
Medication for motion sickness, if you're susceptible
Telephone numbers:
    A travel advisory service with 24-hour hotline
    Local doctors, if available
    The U.S. Embassy
    Your doctor at home

---

nated with the bacterium *Clostridium tetani*, this germ may release a toxin, tetanospasmin, into the bloodstream. Tetanospasmin is one of the most potent toxins known. It affects the nerves going to muscles, freeing the muscles from nervous system control. Muscles can then contract in explosive spasms after the least provocation, a serious situation. When this happens to the facial muscles, it is called lockjaw.

The two things you can do to protect yourself from tetanus are to properly care for all wounds and be sure your immunizations for tetanus are up to date. Tetanus occurs almost exclusively in persons who are unimmunized or inadequately immunized. Not surprisingly, then, it is now rare in the United States, but endemic in developing countries. The shot adults should request to prevent tetanus is called tetanus toxoid. It is abbreviated Td. (It comes combined with diphtheria toxoid—an added benefit.) If you've never received tetanus toxoid, you need a primary series of three injections. Most people, however, just need a single booster if ten or more years have lapsed since their last dose. This is a good idea, whether or not you will be traveling.

Rabies. Any warm-blooded animal can carry and transmit the rabies virus, and many do so without showing any signs of an illness. In the United States, you can generally assume that pets and domesticated animals are properly immunized against rabies. This is not true in many other countries. In most parts of the world, dogs still transmit most cases of rabies. When traveling abroad, the less contact you have with animals the better.

In the United States, we treat for rabies only after someone has a wound of substantial risk, especially one caused or contaminated by a skunk, raccoon, fox, or bat. But if your vocation or avocation is likely to put you in contact with wild or domestic animals overseas, strongly consider getting the rabies vaccine before you go. (It may be hard to get the proper shots while traveling.) The human diploid cell rabies vaccine is administered in three shots into the muscle. Sometimes it is given under the skin, but this method is less effective, especially if you are taking chloroquine for malaria prevention. The pretravel series can be completed in thirty days. If indeed you do sustain an animal bite or a wound contaminated by an animal's saliva, you should still try to get two more shots of the same vaccine. But, because you were vaccinated earlier, the need to get the rabies shots is much less urgent and you have saved yourself from needing a much more extensive series of shots. You will also have no reason to consider taking toxic rabies injections that are still used in some other countries.

Plague. Plague is an often fatal disease that can start in the lymph nodes (bubonic plague) or the lungs (pneumonic plague) and can invade the bloodstream, causing shock. Plague is caused by *Yersinia pestis*, the same bacteria that killed over half the population of Europe in the Middle Ages. (The nursery rhyme "Ring around the rosy"—or rosary—refers to persons dying of plague.) Plague then was transmitted from person to person, but today it is usually carried by rodents—for example, rats, chipmunks, ground squirrels, and hares, and is found in rural, upland areas. If your travel will unavoidably put you in close contact with rodents or rabbits in such an area, anywhere in the world, know your risks well and limit exposure with long clothing, masks, and gloves. Currently, no plague vaccine is available in the United States. Research is in progress, but we are not likely to have vaccines for several years or more.

Plague in its pneumonic form is not a risk for travelers. In 1994, there was a widely publicized epidemic of pneumonic plague in India. Although fifty-three Indian nationals died, no travelers became ill and no plague cases were reported among U.S. residents of India.

Skin-penetrating parasites. There are a number of parasites that can burrow through intact skin, then enter your circulation and cause serious infections. A few of them will occasionally present problems for travelers. These include schistosomiasis, hookworm infections, and strongyloidiasis. Each is a different kind of worm infection.

Schistosomiasis is found widely throughout the world, including large areas of Africa, Arabia, Japan, China, the Philippines, South America, and parts of the Caribbean. There are four different varieties, and symptoms vary, but at its worst, schistosomiasis can lead to liver cirrhosis, bladder cancer, or paralysis.

Hookworm infection is very common in tropical and subtropical zones (between 45 degrees north and 30 degrees south latitude) wherever sanitation is poor. Hookworms will grow in your intestine and spill small amounts of blood every day; patients with hookworms can become quite anemic.

Strongyloidiasis is also distributed widely in the tropics and subtropics. Once established in the intestines, strongyle worms can persist for decades, causing a variety of chronic abdominal problems including pain, nausea, bloating, and diarrhea. If the immune system of a person with strongyloidiasis becomes dysfunctional, the worms can then spread throughout the body, a catastrophic situation.

In many countries, schistosome larvae (which are microscopic worms) might be waiting to strike in fresh water, especially in slow-moving water in rural areas downstream from human habitation. Hookworm and *Strongyloides* larvae attack from soil. So, the methods for preventing these types of infections are simple. As a rule, in areas endemic for schistosomiasis, swim only in salt water; rivers, lakes, and streams are best viewed from the shore. If you need to ford fresh water, be sure you are wearing boots that extend above the water line at all times. Chlorinated swimming pools are safe from these worms.

Heating bath water to 122°F (50°C) for five minutes, or treating it with iodine as you would drinking water, will also help to protect you from schistosomiasis. Wherever you might be at risk for hookworm or strongyloidiasis, simply do not walk barefoot when you are outside.

Several other skin-penetrating parasites can make unsightly and annoying lesions on your skin. The diseases they cause are called cutaneous larva migrans, myiasis, and tungiasis. These parasites will invade no deeper than your skin and therefore won't cause life-threatening illness, but they are worth avoiding nonetheless. Cutaneous larva migrans, commonly known as "creeping eruption," is the most common of these. It occurs all over the world, but mostly in tropical and subtropical countries. In this disease, the hookworm larvae of animals, usually those of dogs, mistakenly penetrate your skin, usually your feet and legs, instead of attacking their intended host. Although the tiny worms cannot mature and reproduce in a human, they will crawl around under your skin producing an extremely itchy, red, twisted trail. Although you can cure creeping eruption easily with a pill called ivermectin, you'll be better off to avoid it in the first place. You do this the same way you avoid human hookworms—don't let unprotected parts of your body contact soil. Creeping eruption can also occur after exposure to sand, so follow the same principle on beaches if you've seen that dogs are around. One in eight cases of creeping eruption occurs on the buttocks and genitals of folks who apparently were nude in the sand on the wrong beaches. The two less common skin-only diseases, myiasis and tungiasis, are also tropical; myiasis occurs when flies deposit their eggs on your skin; tungiasis is caused by a flea. In the rural tropics, if you avoid flies (as much as possible), keep any open wounds or sores properly covered, and do not go barefooted, your chances of getting these infections are minimal.

Hepatitis B. Hepatitis B is a very common disease in other

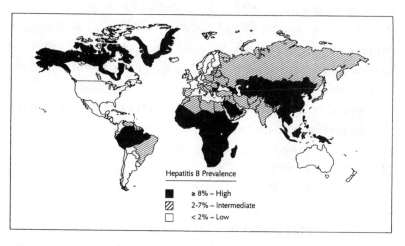

FIGURE 7.3 *Hepatitis B in the world*
SOURCE: Adapted from Centers for Disease Control, *Health Information for International Travel 1993* (Atlanta, Ga.: U.S. Department of Health and Human Services, 1993): 99.

countries (see figure 7.3). It is also the most serious of the different kinds of hepatitis and is hard to treat. It is easy to catch, but only if you have intimate contact with an infected person. If even microscopic drops of an infected person's blood enter tiny breaks in your skin, you can contract hepatitis B. This can happen during sex, but also with sports, camping, certain work projects, military exercises, and the like. If activities involving physical contact with the local population might be part of your plans, and your itinerary includes high-risk areas, get vaccinated before leaving the States. Details about the three-shot series of vaccinations and more information about hepatitis are given in chapter 11.

More ways to keep travel trouble-free

If you have some key medical information—a copy of your last EKG if you have heart disease, for example—carry it with you. Take medications in their original labeled containers; if you are taking any controlled substances, have a doctor's explanatory letter with you.

If you are pregnant, traveling to remote areas is not the best idea. The middle trimester is the safest time to travel because you are least likely then to need the help of an obstetrician. But there are many other problems that can arise. For example, no effective preventive medication for resistant malaria is safe for you during pregnancy, and neither are the best antibiotics for diarrhea. There are many vaccines you will not want to take. Doesn't it make more sense to go another year instead?

Your medical insurance may not cover you when you are in other countries, and reimbursement for a medical evacuation by helicopter and/or airplane is even less likely to be covered. Check your existing medical, auto, and homeowner's insurance and credit card benefits before you leave. If your insurance is inadequate for unforeseen events in foreign countries, get additional coverage. Asking your existing insurance company for a short-term rider is likely to be the least expensive way to get what you need.

Travel agents will offer insurance, but they can charge up to 30 percent of the premium in commission. If you think that you really might need urgent care while away, either because of your medical history or because of your particular travel plans, consider getting insurance from a company that specializes in services for travelers. Two such companies are the Access America Service Corporation (866-807-3982) and International S.O.S. Assistance (215-244-1500). If you are going to pay for this special service, be sure you get access to a 24-hour hotline for advice, local referrals to English-speaking doctors in other countries when needed, and benefits that cover medical evacuation. Be sure to clarify coverage for any preexisting conditions.

Final planning

Start preparing at least one month before travel. There may be a lot to get done for certain trips. Follow the following steps and you'll minimize the odds of coming home with any extra pathogenic baggage.

1. Reread the four general advice sections above about how to avoid travelers' infections that can be contracted from food, insects, air, and skin contact.

2. Review your itinerary and check it against table 7.5 to find out which of the more specific preventive measures—the shots and pills—you need to get before leaving. For additional information, you can turn to the CDC's Web site (www.cdc.gov), the travelers' clinics available in most large cities, and your tour company, if you are using one.

3. Make an appointment with a physician or health clinic to review the immunizations you need, to receive the vaccinations, and to get necessary prescriptions. Unless there is a travelers' clinic in your area, the most expedient way to get what you will need is to see an infectious disease specialist. You could locate one by asking your regular physician, by looking in the phone book, or by requesting a referral through your health plan or a large hospital in your area. The best way to obtain a list of doctors who are knowledgeable about travelers' health is to check with the International Society for Travel Medicine at www.istm.org.

4. Just in case, obtain the names of recommended English-speaking physicians who practice at your destinations. Such a directory is available from the International Association for Medical Assistance to Travelers, 736 Center St., Lewiston, NY 14092.

5. Prepare a travel kit for preventing infection. Suggestions for its contents are listed in table 7.4.

6. Despite your best efforts, you may pick something up during your journey. It happens. Your first symptoms may not

TABLE 7.5
Preventive medicines and vaccines for travelers

Illness	Where you are at risk	When to take the vaccine or medicine . . .
Cholera	Wherever sanitation is suboptimal[a]	No available vaccine
Diphtheria	Worldwide	If it has been 10 years since your last shot
Hepatitis A	Wherever sanitation is suboptimal[a]	If you've never had hepatitis A
Hepatitis B	See figure 7.3	If you will have physical contact with local persons or their blood
Japanese B encephalitis	All Asia	If you're staying over 2 weeks in rural areas during the transmission season
Malaria	See figure 7.1	In all areas of risk
Measles	Worldwide	If you were born after 1957 and not vaccinated after 1980
Meningococcal meningitis	Most of the developing world	Whenever prolonged contact with the local populace is likely
Mumps	Worldwide	If measles vaccine (MMR) is given
Plague	In rural upland areas	No available vaccine
Polio	In nations where polio still exists	One booster in adulthood
Rabies	The developing world	If contact with warm-blooded animals is likely
Rubella	Worldwide	If measles vaccine (MMR) is given
Tetanus	Worldwide	If it has been 10 years since your last shot
Typhoid fever	Wherever sanitation is suboptimal[a]	If you will be eating while off usual tourist routes
Yellow fever	See figure 7.2	In all areas of risk

[a]In most of the world; narrowly, countries considered "developing nations"; broadly, all countries other than the United States, Canada, Japan, Australia, New Zealand, and those of Western Europe.

occur until after you've returned home. The closer to the time of travel, the more likely an illness is related to the trip. However, up to a year could go by before an infection incubating from your trip surfaces. Improper diagnosis can be life threatening if you turn out to be have typhoid fever, amebic dysentery, or malaria. Identify an infectious disease specialist you can see.

You may never be more at risk for contagious diseases than during travel. So it makes sense to spend extra time and organization on prevention.

8   *Pneumonia and Legionnaires' disease*

You may ingest a couple of liters of food and drink in a normal day. However, you exchange gases as you breathe at a rate of more than five liters a minute. Except for our skin, our respiratory tracts are in more contact with our environment than any other part of us. It is no wonder that the most common infections we suffer affect the respiratory tract. Although the germs that cause Legionnaires' disease and many other serious pneumonias do get into our body in the air we breathe, you will find out in this chapter that the germs causing more ordinary pneumonia are already present in the body before the infection starts. Here's how that happens.

Your lungs must remain sterile—unlike your mouth and colon, which normally harbor bacteria. And an elaborate mechanism is at work to keep all kinds of germs out of your lungs. When this system malfunctions, microbes enter your lungs and begin to multiply there. In turn, your body's immune system responds by massing armies of white blood cells in your lungs. The resulting battle leaves behind the corpses of both invading germs and immune cells plus extra body fluids, all of which fill the lung spaces that, in health, contain only air. This inflammatory reaction in the lung is pneumonia.

Pneumonia is both very common and very dangerous. Over three million people develop pneumonia each year in the United States. Twenty-five percent of these patients will have the most serious forms of pneumonia: bacteria will invade their bloodstream. One in five of those people will die, even if they receive the proper antibiotics.

Although eliminating all chance of pneumonia is not possible, you can reduce your risk considerably. In order to do that, you must first understand how your defense mechanisms against pneumonia work, how they might be breached, and when you are at greatest risk.

Bacteria that commonly cause pneumonia reside in the mouth. The lungs start only inches below the mouth. What stops the germs from descending to the lungs? First, whenever you swallow, your vocal cords close off the airway. (Try to swallow and vocalize simultaneously.) Your epiglottis—the flap over the top of your windpipe—provides an additional barrier. If these stopgaps malfunction, you can breathe liquids or solids into your lower airways. This is called "aspiration," and the aspirated materials generally carry bacteria from the mouth with them. Your body quickly recognizes the intrusion and reacts with a violent burst of air that forces the foreign materials back up into your mouth: you cough. However, very small quantities of aspirated material may not elicit a cough reflex. The bacteria in these particles will settle on the mucus that lines the airways. This mucus is constantly moving upward, propelled by small beating hairs (cilia). So bacteria that are caught in the mucus get carried back up the windpipe to the mouth on the "mucociliary ladder."

When pneumonia-causing bacteria do manage to get down into the lungs—after avoiding the epiglottis, the vocal cords, the cough, and the mucus—pneumonia is still unlikely. Waiting in the smaller, lower air sacs of the lungs are antibodies to bind the invaders and white blood cells to engulf them. Occasionally, invading germs can overcome all these immune defenses by their strength of numbers and/or their virulence. Only then will they remain in the lung long enough to multiply and cause disease.

Now that you know how the body blocks bacteria from the lungs, you can easily imagine situations in which pneumonia might occur. If you follow the respiratory tract from the mouth down, you can easily predict conditions that will promote pneumonia: weakness of the muscles of the throat (as in multiple sclerosis), lack of cough (a person on a ventilator or paralyzed from a stroke), an ineffective mucociliary ladder (for example, a rare condition called "immotile cilia syndrome"), or inadequate antibodies in the lung's air spaces (as in immune deficiency diseases). But these are examples of relatively uncommon conditions. There are also much more common reasons why the body's array of defenses against pneumonia may fail.

Smoking is one common reason people may carry extra pneumonia-causing germs in their mouth and upper airways, and thus be at increased risk. Alcohol may be the culprit in as many as a third of all pneumonias. When you are intoxicated, the coordination of your throat muscles is impaired, and aspiration is much more likely to occur. There are many common reasons for an ineffectual cough: for example, rib injuries, in which cough is painful; cancer, in which a tumor may obstruct the flow of air and mucus; and merely the weakness of old age.

Every winter, hospitals overflow with cases of pneumonia associated with influenza. The influenza virus paralyzes the mucociliary ladder and thus permits the pneumonia-causing bacteria to reach the lung. Defects of antibodies and white blood cells are still the least common reason someone might be predisposed to pneumonia. However, the lowered immune response of people infected with HIV makes them vulnerable to bacterial pneumonia.

I have cataloged the conditions that predispose people to pneumonia in table 8.1.

Preventing pneumonia

Pneumonia can be caused by many different bacteria, viruses, occasionally yeasts, and sometimes even parasites. The

TABLE 8.1
Conditions that can predispose you to pneumonia

Mechanism	Common causes	Uncommon causes
Incoordination of throat and vocal cords	Intoxication Head injury Stroke	Seizures Multiple sclerosis
Ineffectual cough	Old age Chest injury	Lung cancer Muscular dystrophy
Paralysis of the mucociliary ladder	Influenza Smoking	Immotile cilia syndrome
Inadequate immune response in the lung or blood	HIV infection	Multiple myeloma Lymphoma Antibody deficiency Organ transplantation

most common organism causing pneumonia is a bacterium, *Streptococcus pneumoniae,* commonly called the pneumococcus. It comes in eighty strains. Therefore, a single vaccine offering absolute protection from pneumonia has not been made. I expect one will never be developed. Nevertheless, you can take several precautions that should greatly diminish the odds of your lungs becoming infected.

Smoking not only promotes growth of common pneumonia-causing bacteria, it also hampers the clearance of bacteria from the airways. It poisons the mucociliary mechanism. People who have smoked for years may develop chronic obstructive pulmonary disease, which is characterized by the production of excessive mucus (chronic bronchitis) and distorted airways and lung cavities (emphysema). These can compound the risk of pneumonia beyond the risk that smoking incurs by itself. Add infection to the long list of reasons not to smoke.

Alcohol—more specifically ethanol—itself is not a risk factor for infection, but intoxication is, no matter what substance you get drunk on. If you are intoxicated, reflexes that close off the airways during swallowing will be out of kilter and the cough reflex will be dulled. If you start vomiting, this carries an additional risk of aspiration. If you follow the ancient Greek credo "Everything in moderation, nothing in excess," you'll go a long way toward avoiding pneumonia.

Another type of pneumonia, anaerobic lung abscess, is caused by aspiration of the bacteria residing in the crevices of the gums and teeth; it occurs only in those with poor dental hygiene and pyorrhea. (It rarely ever happens in persons without teeth.) Here is another reason to brush, floss, and have periodic professional dental cleaning.

Pneumonia most commonly occurs on the coattails of a cold or flu. By avoiding these upper respiratory tract infections, you're helping to prevent pneumonia. So, try to avoid exposure to persons with these infections. Direct contact allows the greatest chance of transmission. You, of course, don't want anyone to cough or sneeze on you, but a hug or a handshake from someone with a cold or flu can pass on the virus just as effectively.

Don't smoke. Avoid excess alcohol. Take care of your teeth and gums. Avoid people with colds and flus. These are admonitions worthy of the most doting mothers or grandmothers. They were right! They didn't want you to wind up in the hospital with pneumonia, and neither do I. However, not all commonly given advice is valid. Now I would like to point out a few things you do *not* need to worry about, so you can concentrate on more important issues.

There is no evidence that getting cold, wet, or cold *and* wet will cause a respiratory illness. The association between bad weather and respiratory bugs is just circumstantial. We tend to be in closer quarters in the winter and it's easier for the viruses to be spread around. I've often wondered whether we link the two because we shiver both when we feel cold and when we are getting a fever. In a similar vein, contrary to early reports, vitamin C (ascorbic acid) does not affect respiratory infections. I think there will always be believers in the efficacy of large doses of vitamin C. They are unlikely to do themselves any good, but most won't harm themselves either. (Vitamin C is toxic only in very high doses; for example, over two grams of vitamin C per day taken regularly may cause kidney stones.)

Vaccines and preventive medications

Of all viral infections, influenza makes you most prone to pneumonia. Influenza is a specific viral infection. There are numerous other respiratory viruses that may cause a flulike illness, but true influenza is an illness caused by influenza viruses A or B. After true influenza, bacterial pneumonia is common and may be severe and life threatening. It is at the end of a week's time, when recovery from influenza is evident, that the pneumonia tends to strike. The pneumococcus is the usual offending germ after influenza, but even more virulent bacteria (such as *Staphylococcus aureus*) become increasingly prevalent.

Influenza occurs every late fall or winter in the United States and takes about six weeks to spread through the community. Each year the severity differs. The most striking example is the influenza epidemic of 1918 in which over 220 million people died worldwide, 500,000 in the United States alone; in a single week that October, 46,000 people died just in Philadelphia. Even now, in the era of antibiotics, catastrophes occur each year. In the most serious forms of pneumonia, antibiotics have little effect during the first four days of treatment. Again, prevention is by far the safest route to travel.

Both a vaccine and medication are available to help you prevent influenza and thereby lessen your chance of pneumonia. Generally, the vaccine is safer, more convenient, and more protective.

Not everyone needs to receive influenza vaccine, but each year many people who should have it don't. The major reason

TABLE 8.2
Side effects of influenza vaccine

Symptom	Frequency	Severity
Soreness at the vaccination site	Common	Mild
Flulike symptoms	Uncommon	Mild
Immediate allergy (to egg protein)	Very rare	Severe

for this may be fear of side effects. Yet, the vaccine is actually very safe (see table 8.2). This vaccine is made up of killed viruses. It is not infectious. It cannot cause influenza. Many people say they've "gotten the flu" from the vaccine and then don't want to take it again. Yes, you can get a low-grade fever and muscle aches for a day or two after this shot, but you are not infected. And since you're not infected, you're not contagious to others and you're not prone to get pneumonia. You can also get a sore arm from a flu shot. It is true that in 1976 there was a batch of swine flu vaccine that caused a rare and serious nervous system disorder (called Guillain-Barré syndrome) in some people who had the shot. This had never happened before and hasn't happened since. It should no longer be a concern. There are very few good excuses for refusing flu shots. If you're one of those rare individuals who are allergic to eggs, though, don't get the shot—the vaccine virus is grown in eggs.

It takes two weeks for influenza vaccine to do its job, and then it lasts only for several months. Taken too late, it might not have time to become effective when the yearly epidemic strikes. The optimal timing for vaccination (most seasons) is around the first of November. If flu arrives early, news reports in October will usually tip you off that you should get the shot that month.

Who should take influenza vaccine? Persons in whom a serious respiratory infection might be catastrophic should definitely be vaccinated. Also, those who in turn might infect high-risk individuals should be vaccinated as well. More specifically, the CDC in Atlanta recommends the following persons receive yearly influenza shots:

- ❏ Persons 50 or older
- ❏ Pregnant women
- ❏ Persons with chronic lung ailments
- ❏ Persons with chronic heart ailments
- ❏ Persons with diabetes
- ❏ Persons with kidney failure
- ❏ Persons with sickle cell disease
- ❏ Immune-deficient persons
- ❏ Medical personnel with patient contact
- ❏ Household members of high-risk persons

If you do not fit into any of these categories, you may still wish to receive the vaccine. Every winter I care for one or two previously healthy individuals who get critically ill from influenza or pneumonia. And I see many more who have their lives disrupted, lose time from work, and just feel miserable.

Influenza viruses are always changing. The prevalent strain one winter is replaced the next. Therefore, a new batch of influenza vaccine has to be made each summer, based on advance notice of strains that are affecting other parts of the world. For this and other reasons, no vaccine is 100 percent effective, but it does make a significant difference. In an average year, taking the vaccine will decrease your chance of getting flu to one-fifth that of an unvaccinated person.

If you are in a high-risk group but can't take influenza vaccine, or if you missed it, you have another option. If the epidemic that year is influenza A, there are two medications you can take that may be very helpful: amantadine (Symmetrel) and rimantadine (Flumadine). These medicines won't work on the B variety, but that's usually milder anyway. Two new flu drugs, oseltamivir (Tamiflu) and zanamivir (Relenza) treat A and B. If you are already on one of these four medicines before being exposed to the virus, it may work as well as the vaccine. If you start it after symptoms begin, it may help make the disease milder, but may or may not help protect you from pneumonia. Influenza vaccine takes two weeks to become effective; if you get vaccinated late, you can stop the treatment after two weeks. If not, take one of these medicines for the full time influenza is going through the community.

No vaccine will render you completely immune to pneumonia, but there is one vaccine that might help. It is called pneumococcal polysaccharide vaccine, or Pneumovax-23. This shot will help protect you from the most common strains of pneumococcus, but not from other pneumonia-causing bacteria, nor the cold or influenza viruses.

Like influenza vaccine, pneumococcal vaccine is most important for those of us at highest risk of getting the disease and/or having a more serious case. Pneumococcal pneumonia occurs most commonly in older adults. If you are over fifty, consider taking the vaccine. It is highly recommended for anyone over sixty-five. Others who benefit include persons infected with the HIV virus; those whose spleens have been removed; persons on dialysis; persons with sickle cell disease; diabetics; people with cardiovascular disease; and anyone else with a predisposition to pneumonia. A booster shot of pneumococcal vaccine should be considered in six years.

Pneumovax-23 is a very safe vaccine. It is made from the outside coatings of twenty-three of the most common strains of pneumococcus that cause disease. It is a killed vaccine. You cannot get infected from it. It will not cause more side effects than a sore arm and a low-grade fever for a day or two. Most recipients have no side effects.

Unusual types of pneumonia

So far, I have suggested to you several personal care measures and two kinds of vaccinations that will go a long way to decrease your chances of coming down with common pneumonia. However, there are many other causes of pneumonia, many of which are quite rare. Since some are eminently avoidable, I would like to point out briefly where these pneumonias are found, how they are contracted, and how to best avoid them. Following that is a larger discussion of one unusual (but not rare), particularly severe pneumonia: Legionnaires' disease.

Brucellosis. You can get brucellosis from animals, in particular, goats, cattle, pigs, and hogs; less often from dogs or sheep; rarely from wild animals. You can pick up *Brucella*, the bacterium that causes brucellosis, by direct contact with the animal or its urine. Meatpackers, farmers, and veterinarians are the most commonly affected. You can also get brucellosis by drinking unpasteurized milk. The disease occurs worldwide. Those at risk should consider wearing protective glasses and clothing whenever they are close to animals. Better yet, be sure the animals have been properly vaccinated for brucellosis. Always avoid raw milk.

Coccidioidomycosis. Also called San Joaquin Valley fever, coccidioidomycosis is most common inland in California, and its incidence there waxes and wanes, for example, there was a surge in Kern County following the Northridge earthquake. But coccidio-idomycosis also occurs in areas of Arizona, New Mexico, Texas, and southern Nevada (see figure 8.1). It is entirely confined to the Americas. The disease is caused by spores of a fungus found in desert soils. Avoid breathing in dusts during dry season in regions where the disease is endemic. Although you can catch this fungus by merely driving though an endemic area, certain situations are particularly to be avoided: dust storms and archeology digs.

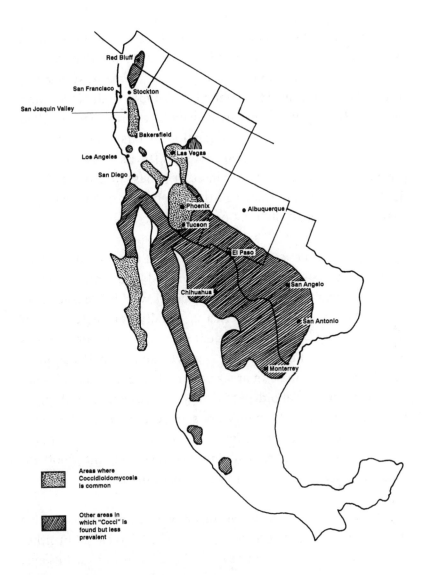

FIGURE 8.1 *Coccidioidomycosis in North America*
The dotted areas are where you can regularly catch "cocci." The hatched areas are where it occurs sometimes.

SOURCE: Adapted with permission from J. N. Galgiani, "Coccidioidomycosis," *Infectious Disease in Clinical Practice* 1 (1992): 357.

Hantavirus pulmonary syndrome. Hantavirus pulmonary syndrome is a newly recognized viral lung disease that can rapidly be fatal. Cases have been diagnosed in many states, but primarily in New Mexico, Arizona, Colorado, Utah, Texas, and Nevada. Hantavirus (primarily caused by a viral species called sinombre) is contracted by inhalation of dusts contaminated with rodent excreta. The deer mouse is the principal reservoir for hantavirus in the United States. It is best to avoid soil and dust aerosols in the deserts of the Southwest or wherever you suspect rodents are living. Control rodents near your home.

Plague. Plague is found in the United States in only fifteen states from Texas, Arizona, Colorado, and Wyoming, and westward. It is also found in selected habitats worldwide (see chapter 7). Plague in North America is usually contracted one of three ways: by flea bite, by rodent bite, or by handling tissues of infected wild mammals. Wear gloves and mask if you must handle wild mammals in areas where plague is endemic. Control fleas on household pets and wear protective clothing in the wild. Squirrels, chipmunks, rats, mice, and prairie dogs may all carry plague. Eliminate food sources for these wild rodents near houses and ensure that your dwelling is rodent proof. For those at unavoidable risk, a vaccine is available.

Psittacosis. All over the world, anywhere people handle live birds, the birdborne infection psittacosis (also called ornithosis or parrot fever) is found. Any bird, even ducks, turkeys, and chickens, can carry and transmit psittacosis, although parrots (including cockatiels) are more likely to do so. In the household, treat any new avian pet with tetracycline for two weeks. This antibiotic is available at any pet store. If you are exposed to birds at work, be sure there is an occupational hazard plan dealing with psittacosis.

Q fever. Q fever is another pneumonia found worldwide and transmitted by livestock. You catch the disease by breathing in infected particles. The vapors created during animal childbirth and emanating from milk are the major risks. Again, don't drink unpasteurized milk. Otherwise, this is an occupational risk of livestock workers, who should be properly instructed by a veterinarian as to safe handling of pregnant cattle, sheep, or goats.

Tularemia. Also called rabbit fever, the bacterial infection tularemia is found only in the Northern Hemisphere. In North America, its range goes from the Gulf Coast north to the Arctic Circle. You can catch tularemia by touching the tissue of an infected mammal, classically by skinning rabbits. Tick bites can also transmit tularemia. Hunters, trappers, and farmers are most likely to contract the disease skinning game. Wear gloves and a mask when you skin game. Prevent tick bites with repellents and by wearing protective clothing. There is currently no vaccine available to protect you from tularemia.

Legionnaires' disease

Legionnaires' disease (or Legionellosis) is another pneumonia caused by a bacterium (*Legionella*). It deserves special attention because, compared to the more common pneumococcal pneumonia, Legionnaires' pneumonia carries a risk of death of up to 30 percent. Furthermore, it does not respond to penicillin or the other antibiotics physicians frequently prescribe for pneumonia. So, prevention is obviously even more important for *Legionella* than for many of the other germs that attack the lungs.

Legionnaires' disease can occur in outbreaks like the infamous one in 1976 that affected 222 people after the American

Legion convention in Philadelphia and the one that sickened 24 people aboard a cruise ship in 1994, but it can also occur sporadically. For example, in a recent survey of one Ohio county, 5 percent of pneumonias treated at community hospitals were Legionellosis. It accounts for 10,000 to 25,000 cases of pneumonia annually in the United States.

The bacteria that cause Legionellosis are common in our environment. You can isolate them in one-third of our homes, one-half of our large buildings, and three-quarters of our hospitals. Nevertheless, the risk of Legionellosis remains low for most people who are not highly susceptible to the germ. The risk of Legionellosis increases substantially, however, in the following groups: the elderly, especially smokers with chronic lung disease; certain persons with malignancies, especially those with lymphoma or a rare disease called "hairy cell leukemia"; those with kidney failure; organ transplant recipients; and people taking cortisone. People in these groups in particular should be alert to situations where *Legionella* bacteria might flourish.

The bacteria that cause Legionellosis thrive in warm fresh water. (They particularly like water with some sediment and at a temperature between 25° and 42°C [75° to 110°F]). You can contract it by inhaling contaminated mists. Cases have been traced to aerosols of shower water (at home or in hospital), drinking water, water in air-conditioning cooling towers, lake water, stream water, humidifiers, whirlpool spas, decorative fountains, and even the mist sprayed over vegetables at supermarkets.

Legionellosis is rare enough that most of us really need not be concerned. However, *for those who are most susceptible*, the following measures can be taken to lower their risk of contracting Legionnaires' disease:

1. Stay clear of cooling towers.
2. Have your home water heater cultured for *Legionella*. If

it turns out to be positive, periodically increase the temperature of your heater water to 60°C (140°F) for several days. This temperature is lethal to the germ. Beware of scalding, which may occur when the water is 52°C (125°F) or more! (A similar but less demanding approach is to let the hot water run for five or ten minutes before you shower, to flush and sterilize the showerhead.)

3. If you must be admitted to the hospital for any reason, ask for a conference with the infection control nurse. Ask if there have been cases of Legionellosis contracted in the hospital. If so, have decontamination procedures been carried out? If you are told that a substantial risk of Legionnaires' disease remains, talk to your physician about the advisability of remaining in that hospital or of taking prophylactic erythromycin—one antibiotic that is effective against *Legionella*.

Three

Infections you get from others

9   *Tuberculosis*

*T*uberculosis (infection with the bacterium *Mycobacterium tuberculosis*) kills more of us around the world than any other infection. About two billion persons harbor this germ, and each year ten million get ill from it. Another three million persons die every year of tuberculosis.

Up to the beginning of the twentieth century, tuberculosis (TB) was the leading overall killer in the United States, but, thanks chiefly to a higher standard of living and better general sanitation, the death rate started to decline and continued to fall through most of the century. When very effective anti-TB antibiotics became available (especially isoniazid, or INH, in 1952), it seemed as if medical science was on the verge of wiping out the dread disease. By the early 1980s, the United States had the lowest tuberculosis rate in its history and the federal Centers for Disease Control set a goal of eliminating tuberculosis "by the year 2010." But TB would not die. To the contrary, in 1985 its incidence began to rise (see figure 9.1).

This unfortunate turnaround may be due to an increase in populations at great risk for TB: people infected with HIV, Asian and Hispanic immigrants, and drug users who inject substances intravenously. Although the upswing has now been checked, plenty of TB remains in the United States.

TB is stealthy. When *Mycobacterium tuberculosis* enters your body, you will notice few or no distinctive symptoms. You might think you have an ordinary cold, flu, or bronchitis; even a medical examination at this stage probably won't detect TB unless the doctor is very alert to the possibility. Typically, the TB germ then spreads through the bloodstream unnoticed, and over the

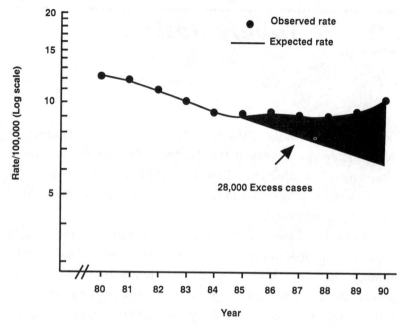

FIGURE 9.1 *Observed versus expected TB cases in the United States*
Source: Adapted from J. A. Jereb, G. D. Kelly, S. W. Dooley Jr., G. M. Cauthen, and D. E. Sinder Jr., "Tuberculosis Morbidity in the United States: Final Data, 1990," *Morbidity and Mortality Weekly Report* 40 (SS–3) (1992): 23.

course of a month (except in infants and persons with poor immune function), the body's white blood cells wall off the invader. The bacteria are engulfed by the white blood cells, which congregate in clusters called granulomas. But the TB germs will persist inside granulomas, living there for many years. At any time later in life the bacteria can begin to multiply again (or "reactivate") and cause disease.

The first two or three years following exposure are the riskiest period for reactivation. The TB bacteria may start reproducing at any time during this period. Later, there is generally some reason for reactivation to occur. Typical reasons include a disease like lymphoma (Hodgkin's disease and others); HIV infection; an immune-suppressing therapy, especially steroids like cortisone; and old age. (As the body ages, and its vigor wanes, that of the immune system does, too.) Each of these factors diminishes the effectiveness of T cells, the kind of white blood cell needed to cordon off TB germs.

Although persons in certain age groups, occupations, nationalities, and living conditions should be especially concerned about TB, every one of us is at some risk. What is your level of risk, and what can you do about it?

The TB skin test

First, find out if you already harbor TB germs. But note that just having the germ inside you does not mean you have tuberculosis. To find out if you've already acquired *Mycobacterium tuberculosis*, ask to take a TB skin test. The best one is known as a PPD, which stands for purified protein derivative. That's what it is—a purified extract of the germ's protein. It is pure and sterile; no one has gotten an infection from this inoculation. The PPD material itself costs less than one dollar per test. It is given free at almost all public health departments; your regular family practitioner, internist, or pediatrician will administer it for a nominal charge.

This is how a PPD test is given. A tiny droplet of PPD (0.1 cc) is injected in the skin on the inside of the left forearm. If the test is done properly, you'll notice a tiny, discrete bump, like that of a small mosquito bite, rise at the site of the test. This bump will quickly flatten and, if TB bacteria have never entered your body, it will stay flat. If, however, you harbor the TB bacillus, your body's immune system will confuse the injected protein with the full bacterium and attempt to wall it off. This takes about two days. Reactions that occur sooner don't count, but at forty-eight to seventy-two hours the PPD result is read.

If the site of the injection is flat, your test is negative. If the site is raised, it should be read by a doctor or nurse. It takes some training and experience to read it correctly. If the raised area is more than 5 millimeters in diameter, you may be tuberculin-positive, or infected with the bacterium. If the raised area is more than 15 millimeters, you are almost certainly infected. Ten millimeters is the most generally accepted cutoff. A common mistake in reading the PPD is to be confused by the area of redness. Even if a large area turns red, the PPD may be normal; only the area of induration (the bump) counts.

There are two more things you should know about TB skin tests. First, the automated types that give multiple little pricks are not as reliable as PPD. They may be more convenient and, if the result reads normal, you can believe it. If there is a reaction, however, you need to confirm it with a PPD. Secondly, the immune system in older people can "forget" how to recognize TB proteins. So individuals over age fifty should be given two PPDs, a week or two apart. The first test is a "reminder" and the second one counts.

Sometimes you will still be asked, usually by an employer, to get a chest x-ray to screen for TB. This is fine—chest x-rays now expose you to very little radiation and give much information. However, you can be infected with TB bacteria and have a normal chest x-ray, while an x-ray that looks like TB can actually represent a handful of other diseases. If you have a normal chest x-ray, you at least know you are not contagious for TB. If you have an abnormal chest x-ray, this will require an evaluation by a medical specialist.

Once you know your PPD status, you may take appropriate action. If you are not infected, you should be in an avoidance mode. You want to dodge situations with potential for spreading TB. If, however, you are already tuberculin-positive, there are certain other steps to take. First, you need to figure out if you have an active case of the disease tuberculosis. If you do, then you need treatment to keep from getting sick and to keep from spreading the disease to other people. If you do not, consider taking preventive medication. I will go over the set of choices you face with each possible PPD status. I will start with the most straightforward of the possibilities.

If you have a negative PPD

You are not ill and are aware of no exposure to TB. Furthermore, you had a skin test and there was no reaction. You know you do not harbor TB and you prefer to remain that way. The most important weapon you have is knowledge. If you understand how transmission occurs, you'll know what situations and places to avoid.

Tuberculosis is transmitted from one person to another. (Transmission from milk or cattle is history in the United States.) TB is spread from person to person by the respiratory route (see figure 9.2). That means it has to make its way from the lungs of an infected person, through the air, and then into the lungs of the next victim. A cough, sneeze, or sometimes even vocalizing can spread the germ from the infected person to the environment.

Another condition is needed, however, for transmission to occur. The germ must make its way to the lowest level of the respiratory tract, stick there, and grow. And for a particle to settle that far, it must be just the right size. Airborne respiratory secretions are not small enough at first. The droplets must evaporate and form "droplet nuclei," which, when inhaled, can make their way completely through the bronchial passages and start a new infection.

Now you know the two requirements for contracting TB: an infected person with communicable disease and the inhalation of droplet nuclei from his or her respiratory secretions. In principle, you know enough to keep yourself from acquiring the disease. In practice, though, you have to be able to (1) recognize who might have communicable TB and (2) avoid spending time with them in poorly ventilated enclosed spaces.

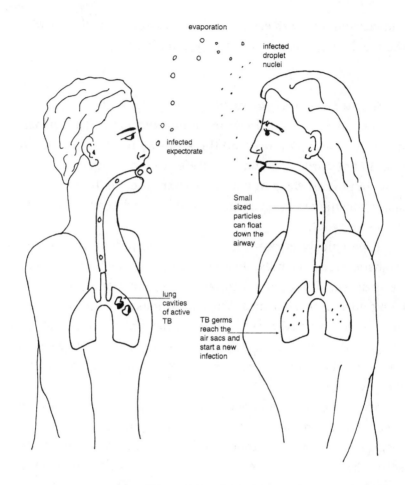

evaporation

infected droplet nuclei

infected expectorate

Small sized particles can float down the airway

lung cavities of active TB

TB germs reach the air sacs and start a new infection

Enclosed space with poor ventilation

FIGURE 9.2   *The transmission of TB*
A person with a tuberculosis lung cavity coughs and contaminates the air in an enclosed space. The infected expectorate dries, becoming droplet nuclei. These are the right size to enter another person's lung and spread TB.

It is well known that someone with advanced TB has a chronic cough, often bringing up blood. This person may also be emaciated. (TB was formerly known as "consumption.") However, the average person with TB does not fit this stereotype, and it is not a simple matter to tell if someone has TB. If you

---

TABLE 9.1
Medical conditions that increase the risk of TB

❏ HIV infection (especially with AIDS)
❏ Previous gastrectomy (partial removal of the stomach for ulcers)
❏ Silicosis (chronic lung disease in quarrymen)
❏ Jejunoileal bypass (bowel surgery for weight loss)
❏ Chronic renal failure (patients on dialysis)
❏ Diabetes mellitus (generally, the insulin-dependent type)
❏ Severe undernutrition (at least 10 percent under ideal weight)
❏ Immune suppressing treatments (especially cortisone or prednisone)
❏ Leukemia or lymphoma (Hodgkin's disease, for one)
❏ Other cancers (especially lung)

---

already know that someone has been diagnosed with tuberculosis, you should avoid being together indoors with that person until he or she has been on a effective therapy for at least two weeks—it takes that long ordinarily to be sure that the disease cannot be spread to you. With the recent spread of resistant TB strains (see below), it may be safer to wait several months to be certain that the treatment has stopped the TB.

If a person has a chronic cough, fever, shaking chills, night sweats, blood spitting (hemoptysis), and/or weight loss, assume the possibility of TB until a doctor proves otherwise. It is more likely to be TB if this person has a medical condition that increases susceptibility to TB (see table 9.1) or if the sick person belongs to a group that is at high risk for the disease (see table 9.2). Then, of course, the odds of the person having or spreading TB go up.

To avoid inhaling droplet nuclei from the infected person's respiratory secretions, the key is ventilation. Outside, there is nothing to worry about. In addition to the breeze sweeping the particles away, the ultraviolet light rays in sunlight are deadly to *Mycobacterium tuberculosis*. Inside, rapid air turnover can make the environment safe. Cross-ventilation with a powerful

---

TABLE 9.2
Groups at high risk for TB

❑ Persons who have resided in high-prevalence areas, such as the Philippines, Southeast Asia, Africa, and much of South America

❑ Medically underserved, low-income, inner-city dwellers, including homeless persons

❑ Residents of nursing homes, mental institutions, and especially prisons

❑ Injecting drug users

---

window fan (blowing to the outside) will do. In places with poorer air flow, it still might take days for you to contract TB from an infected person's coughs, but you would be prudent to avoid any exposure to a potentially infected room. In hospital rooms of patients with suspected or proven TB, a mask and rapid air turnover are now required to reduce the risk of exposure for doctors, nurses, and other staff.

North Americans rarely need to be concerned about crowds at shopping malls, baseball games, and other public areas. Infected individuals don't generally stay long enough to contaminate such places, and ventilation in these areas is often adequate. In certain public institutions—homeless shelters, prisons, and nursing homes, for example—that are inhabited, rather than just visited by people, you should be wary. Still, TB is most often contracted at home.

Tuberculosis is much more common in the developing world than in North America. If you travel to the Philippines, Southeast Asia, and, particularly, Africa, you'll find rates of TB that are well over ten times the rate in the United States. On such trips, follow the avoidance principles more stringently. Get off a bus promptly if someone is coughing, and stay only briefly in enclosed public spaces.

If your PPD is negative, you have one more option. Although not widely known or used much in the United States, there is a vaccine to prevent TB. It is called BCG, which stands for Bacille Calmette-Guérin. (It was developed in France back in 1921.) It is made of bacteria that are close cousins of *Mycobacterium tuberculosis*, but have been bred to be harmless. An inoculation of these bacteria starts a local infection, easily contained by the body. Then you develop an immunity to the vaccine bacteria. Since the immune system does not distinguish between the two "relatives," it will attack *Mycobacterium tuberculosis* as well.

If BCG were truly great, we'd all take it. Unfortunately, it doesn't work all that well. In one study in southern India in the 1970s, it didn't seem to work at all! Most TB specialists believe, however, it can offer 60 to 80 percent protection, at least in children and young adults. The young respond better to BCG than their elders. Two other things factor into the decision to use it or not. First, vaccination with BCG will turn the PPD skin test positive, so you can no longer use the test as a monitor. Second, there is some risk stemming from the vaccine itself. The material in BCG is living microorganisms. Although the virulence of the bacteria is attenuated and normal people can easily contain it, in people with impaired immune systems (people with HIV, for example), the vaccine could cause a disseminated infection. This is wryly called "BCG-osis."

So, who should receive BCG? The answer is not always clear cut. You should consider getting vaccinated with BCG if you are young, have an intact immune system, *and* you can't avoid exposure to TB. For example, if you work in a prison, homeless shelter, or in Africa, or a member of your family has an active case of TB with a resistant strain, consider taking BCG.

If you've been exposed to TB

You may realize that, despite your best efforts, you have been exposed to tuberculosis bacteria. Typically, your source of exposure will be someone in your family. Don't panic! Most persons with TB are not really able to spread the disease to others, and most exposures don't actually lead to transmission. Moreover, if caught early, *Mycobacterium tuberculosis* infection does not usually become the disease tuberculosis.

Your first cautionary step, if you believe you have been exposed, is to find out if you already have TB. Fever, chills, cough, night sweats, shaking chills, and weight loss are the usual symptoms of active tuberculosis, but they're often not dramatic or overwhelming. Whatever the symptoms, you should be seen by a physician no more than three days after exposure. Besides having a physical examination, be sure a chest x-ray is done. If tests show active tuberculosis, you will need treatment. This book is about prevention, not treatment, but suffice it to say that your physician will want to start you on at least three different antibiotics at once.

If you prove not to have active TB, you still could be incubating the disease. The incubation period for TB varies from weeks to decades. That provides an important window of opportunity for prevention. You and your physician need to ask the following questions: First, was your exposure substantial? In other words, were you around someone with known active TB in the lungs? Second, was your contact in the household or another confined space? You or your physician may need to gather information to answer the first question, but the second only takes reflection. If you can answer no to either question, stop worrying and do nothing.

If, however, you had a significant exposure, here are some suggestions to prevent illness: Have a PPD test immediately, and repeat it in six and twelve weeks. If it converts to positive, you are at substantial risk for TB and should start preventive medication. (I will discuss the use of this medicine below.) After exposure, even a 5-millimeter PPD reaction is regarded as significant. Certain groups of individuals are at such great risk of getting TB and, moreover, getting a bad case of it, that they should start the medicine promptly: children under five,

HIV-infected persons, and others whose immune systems are severely compromised. They shouldn't even wait for a positive PPD.

If you have a positive PPD

If the bump produced by a tuberculin skin test is 10 millimeters across or larger, you may have been infected in the past, but you still are very unlikely to have the disease tuberculosis. A physical exam and chest x-ray will be needed to exclude active disease. If these are negative, however, you remain at risk, and active tuberculosis can often be prevented.

The 10-millimeter cutoff is not a precise one. It can't be; humans and bacteria are complex, and biology is not an exact science. On the human side of this equation, not everyone's immune system is functioning up to speed. On the bacterial side, there are many other bacteria related to *M. tuberculosis* that may cause some reaction to PPD, too. All this needs to be considered and weighed in the decisions on how to proceed.

The major question for persons with reactive TB skin tests and no active disease is whether to take a medication called isoniazid (INH) as a prophylactic. In its favor, it works. Against it, you may have to keep taking it for months, and it may be toxic. Taken faithfully, INH can prevent TB in over 90 percent of cases. But potential toxicities include inflammation and injury to the liver and the nerves (hepatitis and neuritis). Blood test monitoring and vitamin B_6 can minimize these risks. (The best set of recommendations regarding when to use INH is outlined in table 9.3.)

INH is taken once daily in pill form. A nine-month course of INH is generally sufficient. However, if there's enough infection to be visible on a chest x-ray, or if your immune system is deficient, stay with it for at least twelve months.

The two main toxicities of INH can easily be avoided. First,

TABLE 9.3
Preventive use of INH against TB

You should consider taking prophylactic INH . . .

❏ *If you are under 35 and basically healthy*
with a PPD of at least 15 mm.

> The 15-millimeter (mm) cutoff decreases false-positive PPDs. INH toxicity is age dependent and unusual in individuals under 35.

❏ *If you are under 35 and in a group with a high prevalance of TB*
with a PPD of at least 10 mm.

> In these individuals a 10-mm reaction is much more likely to mean the real thing. Persons in this category are listed in table 9.2.

❏ *If you are a person with a medical condition that increases TB risk*
with a PPD of at least 10 mm.

> These are conditions that up the ante. They increase the likelihood of getting TB, and some diminish the PPD reaction, so 10 mm gain more importance. These conditions are listed in table 9.1.

❏ *If you are HIV-positive*
with a PPD of at least 5 mm.

> Persons infected with the HIV virus are at great risk for TB and much less likely to react to tuberculin. Five mm are very significant and some patients with no reaction at all should be treated (see chapter 14).

❏ *If you are a person whose chest x-ray suggests old TB*
with a PPD of at least 5 mm.

> The chest x-ray sometimes suggests healed TB; in this case, even a 5-mm reaction usually means *M. tuberculosis* infection. Also, if there's enough infection to show up, the risk of reactivation is higher.

❏ *If you are a recent skin test converter (within 2 years) and under 35*
with a PPD increase of at least 10 mm.

> The risk of becoming ill with TB is greatest in the first two years after acquiring it. "Converter" means increasing by at least 10 mm and going from less than 10 to more. An example would be a college student who had a 3-mm reaction as a freshman and 16-mm reaction as a sophomore.

❏ *If you are a recent skin test converter (within 2 years) and over 35*
with a PPD increase of at least 15 mm.

> With the higher chance of side effects, an increase of at least 15 mm is used to be sure the reaction represents a truly positive test.

SOURCE: adapted from: CDC, "The Use of Preventive Therapy for Tuberculosis Infection in the United States: Recommendations of the Advisory Committee for Elimination of Tuberculosis," *Morbidity and Mortality Weekly Report* 39, RR-8 (1990): May 18, 1990.
NOTE: These are the recommendations of the CDC and the American Thoracic Society.

the neuritis—damaged nerves—only happens in individuals deficient in vitamin B$_6$ (pyridoxine). A small amount, only 10 milligrams per day, prevents neuritis. Pyridoxine can be taken right along with the INH. People over fifty especially need to take it. Second, the hepatitis can be predicted by a blood test, and therefore avoided. The blood test checks levels of a liver enzyme, ALT (formerly called SGPT). If it goes over five times the normal value, stop INH. If you are under thirty-five, your chance of INH hepatitis is under 0.3 percent and you need not check the ALT regularly. Over thirty-five, have it checked at two, four, six, and eight weeks into therapy, and then monthly. If you are taking INH and experience nausea, vomiting, loss of appetite, jaundice (yellowed eyes and complexion), or other-wise become concerned about your liver, stop the drug promptly and contact your physician. In fact, if you have a significant liver disease beforehand, you may not want to take INH. Al-though not totally restricted, alcohol consumption should be kept to a minimum while you're on INH; if you don't think you can do that, you had better not take INH.

And now, the bad news . . .

We can no longer assume that INH will always prevent TB. Indeed, we can no longer assume there are effective antibiot-ics for all strains of TB. In the 1990s we are seeing the rise of multidrug-resistant tuberculosis.

Multidrug-resistant tuberculosis is TB caused by a strain of *M. tuberculosis* that is resistant to INH and to at least one other usual TB drug. Worse, some strains are resistant to all currently available agents. In other words, although it is rare as of this writing, incurable tuberculosis now exists.

To date, multidrug-resistant TB has been largely limited to HIV patients in institutional settings, in New York City (where the rate of resistant TB runs about 20 percent now), its environs (especially Jersey City), and in Miami. Persons with HIV infection catch multidrug-resistant TB infection very easily and, in them, the incubation period is abbreviated and the mortality extraordinary. Three-quarters of the patients in these sad circumstances die in four to sixteen weeks.

Do healthy citizens need to worry about multidrug-resistant TB? Generally, not yet. However, if you do need to take prophylactic medication, and you think you might have acquired an INH-resistant strain, you should receive a drug called rifampin instead. As INH resistance is very common in Vietnam and the Philippines, individuals who originally acquired their TB in these countries should also be treated with rifampin.

Let the resurgance of TB in the U.S. and the growing antibiotic resistance of the TB germ be a wake-up call for us to practice careful prevention.

10 *Sexually transmitted diseases*

Sexual acts may transmit life-threatening diseases. This has been true throughout human history—with the brief exception of about forty years in the middle of the twentieth century. The advent of penicillin in 1941 as treatment for syphilis and gonorrhea led many people to believe that at last medical science could cure sexually transmitted infections. That was an overly optimistic hope. The dramatic spread of the human immunodeficiency virus (HIV) has shown that sexually transmitted diseases (STDs) still pose mortal threats.

Unfortunately, many Americans still have an "it can't happen to me" attitude about sexually transmitted diseases. But it can, whether you are single or married; live in the city, suburbs, or country; are rich, middle-class, or poor; young or old; well educated or illiterate. If you have sex, you put yourself at some risk of catching a sexually transmitted disease. The stakes may be highest with HIV infection; but, even setting HIV aside for a moment, other STDs have to be taken seriously. They are not just inconveniences that can be remedied by a shot of antibiotics.

For example, there is no way to get rid of the viruses that cause genital herpes or genital warts: once you are infected, those viruses stay with you for the rest of your life. The genital wart virus has been associated with cervical cancer. A chlamydia infection may show no symptoms at first but will later cause chronic long-term medical problems, and often infertility. Similarly, an unsuspected syphilis infection can lead to dementia many years later. With many STDs, even if you don't realize you are infected, you can still transmit them to other people. Children may be born with STDs. Some STD infections substantially increase your chances of also acquiring HIV.

Clearly, the best thing to do about STDs is to avoid them. Dealing with them after infection is much harder than preventing them in the first place. In this chapter, I will first explain how you can avoid picking up STDs. In most cases, I'll also tell how they can be treated after exposure but before the disease develops, and, in some cases, how to keep acquired STDs quiescent.

A *universal approach to prevention*

Many different kinds of microorganisms cause STDs—strains of viruses, bacteria, and protozoa—but fortunately, the basic techniques that protect you against one will protect you against others as well.

The one sure way to avoid sexually transmitted diseases is not to have sex. Beyond abstinence, there is always some chance of acquiring an STD during sex, although sometimes the risk is quite low. The risk is related to the choice of partner and the sexual acts performed.

In a long-term monogamous relationship with a person who is faithful, never used intravenous drugs, and has a negative blood test for HIV and syphilis, the risk of acquiring an STD is very small. (The standard premarital blood test is for syphilis.) But each time you encounter a new partner, you have a chance of contracting any STD he or she may have picked up from any previous sexual encounter. If you have sex with lots of different people whom you barely know, your risk (and theirs) of getting infected with an STD is tremendously high.

The acts performed during sex also present a hierarchy of risk. Caressing and hugging are safe even if your partner is

HIV-positive. Ordinary kissing and mutual masturbation are also unlikely to spread an STD, while deep French kissing, kissing if your partner has any gum or mouth sores, and oral-genital sex all increase the risk of exposure to an STD. Unprotected vaginal intercourse with a new and/or unknown partner is highly risky business these days, and unprotected anal intercourse is at least five times worse. Any single sexual exposure might be the one that gives you HIV, herpes, chlamydia, or another STD. And usually there is no way to know beforehand that your partner carries an STD. You have to act on the assumption that he or she does.

If you find yourself in a situation that I have defined as chancy, and you want to proceed anyway, plan ahead enough to keep a barrier between yourself and the secretions (semen and vaginal secretions, but also saliva and blood) of your partner. No matter what your level of respect and affection is for that partner, you don't know what pathogens are in those secretions. This barrier equipment—chiefly male condoms—must be readily available, even in the heat of passion. Take the trouble ahead of time to have the condoms ready at hand in the appropriate bedside drawer, wallet, pocketbook, or glove compartment. One nurse made herself an elegant set of dangling earrings that were actually well-disguised wrapped condoms.

Of all the available barrier methods, so far only the male latex condom has been proven to be an effective barrier to gonorrhea, herpes, hepatitis B virus, chlamydia, and HIV. The latex condom is regulated by the Food and Drug Administration: each condom is tested electronically for holes before packaging. Although it is well known that the condoms are not perfect, they are quite good. Either due to the fault of the devices or their users, condoms do break, but less than 2 percent of the time. They will slip off during intercourse less than 1 in 200 times; the rate of slippage during withdrawal is the same. If you are going to depend on condoms, consistent and correct usage is essential. Consistent usage depends on availability and your personal motivation. Correct usage is easy. Here are the rules:

1. Be sure the container and wrapping are undamaged.
2. Apply the condom after the penis is erect but prior to any genital contact.
3. Leave a small airspace at the tip if one is not built in.
4. Roll the condom all the way to the base of the penis.
5. Ensure adequate lubrication. If this doesn't happen naturally, use a water-based lubricant such as K-Y Jelly.
6. Never allow an oil-based lubricant to touch the condom; these can dissolve latex. Therefore, do not apply massage oils, vegetable oils, shortening, mineral oil, or petroleum jelly.
7. Hold the condom to the base of the penis on withdrawal.
8. Use a new condom with each sexual act.

No other barrier method is reliable as the sole means of preventing STDs. The female condom (Reality) is a sheath with a ring at one end that fits over the cervix. This device has not been systematically tested for STD prevention, but it is not completely reliable for birth control. Over a one-year trial of the female condom, 11 percent of the women who used it for contraception became pregnant. (The rate of pregnancy as the result of failure of the male condom is closer to 1 percent per year.) The diaphragm cervical cap is physically a less effective barrier than any kind of condom, and doesn't protect the vagina or labia at all.

The diaphragm must be used with a spermicide to prevent pregnancy. Spermicides—birth control creams, jellies, and foams—generally contain a substance called nonoxynol-9 as the active ingredient. This substance, even alone, decreases (but does not eliminate) transmission of gonorrhea and chlamydia, and it is quite toxic to *Trichomonas* as well. However, although nonoxynol-9 kills HIV in the test tube, when it was tested in humans, it did not stop transmission of the virus. Moreover, some researchers feel that since the spermicide can injure the vaginal lining it might even increase the transmission of HIV. Nonoxynol-9 alone should not be relied upon to prevent STDs.

Alcohol and drugs are clearly associated with transmission of sexually transmitted disease. If you use drugs or drink, especially if you do so with your sexual partner, take extra forethought about having condoms ready. The chances of remembering while you're high are pretty slim.

It is reasonable to be concerned that the germs that cause STDs might survive in the environment if conditions were right. You might worry about picking up a disease that is usually sexually transmitted at a hot tub, swimming pool, or public toilet if anyone preceding you there was infected. Fortunately, medical scientists have tested those sites and found no evidence of STD transmission.

Disease symptoms and prevention

If you can comply with the generic guidelines given up to this point in the chapter (and listed in table 10.1), you're unlikely to contract any STD. However, each of kind of infection has its own peculiarities. Here is a short description of each major STD (in alphabetical order) with specific advice on how to avoid it.

Chancroid. Chancroid is unusual in the United States (only five thousand cases per year) but common in tropical and subtropical countries. So, you are at risk for chancroid after unprotected sex with someone in those countries or with someone who might have brought it back from overseas. Chancroid is caused by a bacterium, *Hemophilus ducreyi*, and causes a ragged and painful genital sore that may be confused with an injury.

TABLE 10.1
Universal guidelines for preventing sexually transmitted diseases

1. Only have unprotected sexual intercourse (that is, without using a male latex condom) if you know that your partner
   Is your only sexual partner and is faithful
   Was never an injecting drug user
   Has a negative test for HIV (drawn 6 months after their last unprotected exposure to someone else)
   Has no undiagnosed genital problems, including no visible genital sores, rashes, discharges, or other symptoms

2. For all other sexual contacts involving any penetration of any body cavity (mouth, vagina, anus), use a male latex condom properly and consistently.

3. Ordinary kisses are safe, but deep (French) kissing partners should meet the same criteria as listed in number 1.

4. Considered safe without extra precautions: hugging, caressing, fondling, and mutual masturbation.

The sore shows up on the genitals two to five days after exposure. If the disease goes untreated, large swollen groin glands may occur in another week. Since the disease is rare, misdiagnosis is fairly common. If you learn that you have been exposed to a case, seek treatment (with erythromycin, azithromycin [Zithromax], or ceftriaxone [Rocephin]), even if no symptoms have shown up.

Chlamydia. Chlamydia trachomatis is currently causing a silent epidemic. The CDC estimates that four million new *Chlamydia trachomatis* infections occur each year in the United States. Chlamydia is currently most prevalent in young people, particularly in adolescent females, but anyone can carry it. Overall, about 15 percent of sexually active women and 10 percent of sexually active men are infected with chlamydia in the United States. But although it is a very common STD, half the infected persons (who are mostly female) are not even aware that they have a problem.

When chlamydia does cause symptoms, the most noticeable of these are a grayish penile discharge in men, a scant vaginal discharge in women, and some burning on urination. Though the initial symptoms of this bacterial infection may be minor or nonexistent, the disease has to be taken seriously. Left untreated it can cause serious problems: women may experience chronic pelvic pain, infection of the deep pelvic organs (pelvic inflammatory disease), infertility, and ectopic pregnancy. In the course of childbirth, it can infect a newborn's eyes and lungs. Men may develop a painful infection in the scrotum (epididymitis) or chronic arthritis (Reiter's disease).

If you have had any unprotected sex with any new partners, get tested for chlamydia. The tests for it these days are simple and painless and, for a woman, can be part of a routine pelvic exam. If you are informed that you've been exposed, it is not necessary to get tested. Just get treated. Generally, a tetracycline drug (doxycycline) for a week or a single dose of azithromycin (Zithromax) is given, but pregnant women should take only amoxicillin or erythromycin, and later be retested. All your sexual partners must be treated as well, both to prevent illness and to prevent "STD ping-pong," the passing of sexually transmitted diseases back and forth between partners.

Gonorrhea. Referred to in medical lingo as GC, the gonococcus bacterium infects over a million people per year in the United States alone. Like chlamydia, gonorrhea is most commonly a disease of young adults. Unlike chlamydia, its symptoms are usually noticeable, especially in men. Only 10 percent or so of infected men carry gonorrhea without knowing it.

If you are exposed, you will probably get "clap" or "drip" in just a day or two: a painful thick yellow discharge from the penis or vagina. GC can also occasionally affect other parts of the body, causing rash, arthritis, and rarely, more serious infections of vital organs. Men may get a painful scrotal infection called epididymitis and women may get pelvic inflammatory disease.

If you think you've been exposed, get tested. If you know you've been exposed, get treated. These days, a shot is no longer required. A single dose of a pill, usually gatifloxacin (Tequin) 400 mg or ciprofloxacin (Cipro) 500 mg, is all that is needed to prevent or cure uncomplicated GC. However, these bacteria become resistant to whatever is in common usage, as they have to penicillin. When they learn to evade our current treatments, let us hope we've devised some new ones.

Persons who become infected with GC commonly pick up chlamydia simultaneously. This occurs 15 to 25 percent of the time in heterosexual men and 35 to 50 percent of the time in women. The best approach is to automatically get treatment for chlamydia if you need treatment for gonorrhea.

Herpes. There are two types of herpes (or HSV, for herpes simplex virus). HSV type 1 causes the common fever blister, found along the lips or at the cracks of the mouth, often following sun exposure or on the heels of another infection. HSV type 2 is the usual cause of genital herpes.

Herpes viruses, once contracted, stay with you for life. They migrate to the nerve cells next to the spinal cord. The viral DNA is incorporated into the nuclei of your own cells without injuring those cells. There is no known way to eradicate the virus at this point. After certain stimuli, the virus will travel down the nerve cells, back to the skin, and grow there, causing a flare-up. HSV-1 tends to cause flare-ups around the mouth and HSV-2 on the genitals. If you get infected with HSV-1 on the genitals (from oral-genital sex or from your own hands) it can cause infection there once, but won't usually recur. The opposite scenario is similar; HSV-2 tends not to recur on the mouth.

Many people are distraught when they find they have genital herpes. If you are one of them, it may help to know that you are not alone. Genital herpes is a very common infection. According to data from blood tests, thirty million Americans have it, although many may not realize it. Most of the time HSV-2 will cause small clusters of blisters that soon become open sores. They occur anywhere on the male or female genital area and may be painful. Genital herpes is generally worst the first time the symptoms appear. The disease then tends to recur with no obvious reason for its reappearances. However, many atypical lesions may go unrecognized and may be confused with just a minor injury or irritation. The most common time of life to first get HSV is in the twenties, but it can happen at any age.

Three-quarters of the persons infected with HSV-2 will have a recurrence, but often only one. A few (about 10 percent) will have frequent (monthly) recurrences. The risk of frequent flare-ups is one reason not to want to ever get genital herpes. Another is that an infected mother can pass the virus on to her infant as the baby passes through the birth canal (see chapter 15 for details). Genital herpes makes it easier to catch HIV. Finally, if you don't have genital herpes, you cannot spread it to anyone else.

You get genital HSV by having direct contact with someone else who is shedding the virus. Most of the time, that person will have a visible lesion. There is an 80 to 90 percent chance of getting herpes after having sex with someone who has an active lesion. But occasionally you can also contract herpes from someone who does not know they are contagious. The infectious lesion may be insignificant or ignored: it may be out of view (for example, on a woman's cervix); or the person can be shedding virus in otherwise normal secretions. In married couples, if one member is positive and the other is not, there is a 12 percent chance per year of passing on HSV-2.

The best thing you can do to prevent yourself from getting genital herpes is to follow the general guidelines given at the start of this chapter. If you are having unprotected sex in a stable, monogamous relationship, you still run some risk of contracting the virus. If you avoid all direct sexual contact when your partner has any lesions that can be seen or felt, you decrease your risk by a factor of seven. Any lesion counts; even a remnant scab can be infectious. Since herpes, although incurable, is treatable, this approach is reasonable.

Genital herpes is easily controlled with medication. A good drug currently is acyclovir (Zovirax). Although it does not rid you of the viral DNA hiding in nerve cells, it works quite well on the skin lesions. There are two approaches to the use of acyclovir: episodic and prophylactic. Take acyclovir episodically if your outbreaks are only occasional. This way you won't need to be on medicine constantly. Many persons get abnormal sensations—often described as a tingling—before the rash appears and can start the medication at the very earliest stage of an outbreak.

Taken promptly in doses of 200 mg five times daily or 400 mg three times daily for five days, acyclovir can shorten outbreaks to just a day or two at a time. For those with frequent outbreaks, continuous acyclovir use—200 mg three times daily or 400 mg twice daily—is 95 percent effective in preventing recurrent HSV-2. The daily dose of acyclovir should be taken for a year at a time; after that, try going without the medication and see if you still need it. Your recurrence frequency may have dwindled by then, as it tends to do over time. No serious side effects have been reported for either the long-term daily use or occasional use. Although, so far, birth defects have not been associated with acyclovir, it is prudent not to conceive a child while taking it or to take it during pregnancy.

Lice. Pubic lice ("crabs") are contracted during sex. If you notice them on pubic hair you can eradicate them with an over-the-counter preparation: piperonyl butoxide (RID). Apply the shampoo and wash it off after ten minutes. Then immediately use the nit comb that comes with it. To prevent another exposure to these parasites, wash bedding and clothing in a hot cycle in a washing machine and dry clean the blankets and clothes, as necessary. Fumigating is not required. If the lice get on your eyelashes or eyebrows, suffocate them with an occlusive ointment (Vaseline will do) twice daily for ten days. (Head lice are a totally different species of parasite and not an STD.)

Lymphogranuloma venereum. Usually referred to as LGV, lymphogranuloma venereum is another kind of chlamydia. LGV is really quite rare in the United States. It usually is first noticed as tender, enlarged glands on one side of the groin. You won't get LGV if you follow the general guidelines for preventing STDs. Treatment is available with antibiotics, usually tetracycline.

Syphilis. The incidence of syphilis has generally been rising, even in the era of safe sex. Over 100,000 new cases per year are reported in the United States, and thousands of newborns get the infection from their mothers annually (see chapter 15). Although much of the surge in syphilis cases may relate to sex between inner-city injecting drug users and the crack cocaine epidemic, the problem is widespread.

Syphilis is a bacterial infection caused by *Treponema pallidum*, a kind of spiral-shaped bacteria known as a spirochete. It can show up in many different ways. Early on, about one week after infection, it may cause an open but painless genital sore (a chancre). Later, a rash, mouth sores, and swollen glands are common. After many years, if untreated, syphilis can cause dementia, strokes, loss of sensations, leaking heart valves, and hearing loss. Between these various stages, it may be detectable only by blood tests and is said to be latent.

To prevent syphilis, start by following the general guidelines for preventing STDs. The blood test for syphilis can only detect the disease after three months have passed since you were exposed to the spirochete. So, if you suspect you were exposed within the last three months, seek preventive treatment right away. A single shot of benzathine penicillin G (Bicillin LA) 2.4 million units will prevent illness from occurring in the first place. If you are allergic to penicillin (and not pregnant), request doxycycline (Vibramycin) 100 mg by mouth twice daily for two weeks instead.

If you think your exposure to the infection happened more than three months earlier, get tested at your doctor's office or at the health department; by then blood tests will tell you if you've contracted syphilis or not. A screening test, usually one called RPR, is done first. If the screening test is negative, you can trust you do not have syphilis. However, there are many things that make screening tests for syphilis falsely positive, so don't fret if your initial test suggests that you have the disease. (The same is true when this test is run before marriage licenses are granted.) Positive screening tests must be confirmed with a second more specific test, usually called the FTA-ABS. If the confirmatory test is positive, get treatment to protect yourself and others.

Trichomoniasis. The protozoan (one-celled parasite) *Trichomonas* causes a type of vaginitis that is sexually transmitted. It causes a vaginal discharge that is usually frothy, yellowish or greenish, odorous, and associated with genital irritation and burning on urination.

Most of the time vaginitis is not an STD. The garden-variety nonspecific vaginitis and *Candida* (yeast) vaginitis are not. But *Trichomonas*, or "trich" (pronounced trick) for short, is. Any woman treated for vaginitis should ask whether the type of vaginitis she has is *Trichomonas* and whether it could have been contracted sexually. Men carry *Trichomonas* but usually have no symptoms from it; only one in ten will have some discharge from the penis. If you are treated for *Trichomonas*, insist that your sexual partner be treated at the same time so you do not give the infection to each other (or to other partners) again.

Genital warts. Genital warts are caused by the human papilloma virus (HPV). The problem is widespread. In fact, it is the most common STD. If careful testing is done, evidence of HPV can be found in over 25 percent of sexually active women. Over two-thirds of the sexual partners of persons with genital warts will be infected and will usually develop warts about three months after exposure.

Most people with HPV do not know it—either because the warts are hard to see or because the virus has not yet triggered the growth of warts. Only with special testing during a genital exam can it be shown that HPV is present. When the warts do develop, they appear as fleshy clusters of small growths anywhere in the genital region, flat-topped or cauliflowerlike. Although these lesions are generally not painful, they can be disfiguring, and, occasionally, newborns of mothers with genital warts can develop warts on their vocal cords.

Since the only known treatments (various means of surgical removal or interferon injections) merely control these growths but do not eradicate the virus, this is another strong reason you will want to follow the guidelines for preventing STDs. If you find you have been exposed, without protection, to genital warts, unfortunately there's nothing to do or take to prevent problems. Because HPV has been strongly associated with cancer of the cervix, women infected with HPV should be especially careful to get a yearly PAP smear to detect cervical cancer early.

TABLE 10.2
Tests to verify presence of sexually transmitted diseases after exposure

Disease	Test	Timing
AIDS	HIV antibodies	Baseline, 12 weeks, and 6 months
Syphilis	RPR, STS, or VDRL	Baseline, and 12 weeks
Gonorrhea	Culture or antigen	Anytime
Chlamydia	Culture or antigen	Anytime after 1 week
Hepatitis B	HbSAg	Baseline, and 3 months

Because all the diseases in this chapter pass from person to person in essentially the same way, you might wonder if more than one of them can be transmitted at once. The answer is yes, absolutely. So if you pick up any STD, you should get yourself tested for the others. If your partner has already been tested for the range of STDs, this narrows the possibilities of diseases you might have contracted, and you may only need one test or one therapy. However, if you contract an STD and your partner is not fully tested or is unavailable, you might have picked up any number of the diseases in the universe of STDs. In that case, there are certain tests you will want to have run on yourself in order to determine what treatments you need. The studies to have done are listed for you in table 10.2. Use it as a checklist.

11   *Hepatitis*

Hepatitis is frightening. You can contract hepatitis unwittingly. It can make you sick for months. Once infected, you might carry it for life and can pass it to sexual partners and to children at birth. No good treatment for hepatitis is available. Hepatitis can lead to liver failure and liver cancer. Fortunately, it is quite preventable.

Hepatitis is an inflammation of the liver that can be caused by a variety of agents. Viruses are the most common cause, but alcohol, poisons, and medicines cause their share of cases as well. Regardless of cause, all kinds of hepatitis are the same in two respects: First, they all harm the liver and produce essentially the same set of symptoms. Secondly, almost every known cause of hepatitis can be avoided. Unfortunately, each year over fifty thousand new cases of hepatitis are reported to the U.S. Public Health Service. Doubtless, countless more cases go unreported. Evidently, many people are unaware of how to protect themselves from hepatitis. I want to change that.

If you develop hepatitis, your illness is fairly predictable. At first, symptoms would be vague and nonspecific. For days to weeks you might experience only fatigue, low-grade fever, mild nausea, and loss of appetite. Later, your liver might swell and cause discomfort in the right, upper abdomen, especially when jostled. Then, when bile stalls on its passage through the liver, you would likely see dark urine, light stools, and jaundice (yellowing of the skin). When this occurs, you may look worse but actually feel better. Appetite returns, fever and nausea go away, and strength gradually returns.

Although this illness, called "acute hepatitis," is not pleasant

TABLE 11.1
Salient features of hepatitis

Type	Important features	Common means of spread
A	Rarely fatal Never chronic	Contaminated food Contaminated water Close contact with a case
B	Deadly in 1% 10% adults become chronic 50% children get chronic 90% infants are chronic	Close contact with a case Illicit intravenous drugs During childbirth
C	Often becomes chronic	Blood transfusion Illicit drugs
D	Infects only those already infected with B	Illicit intravenous drugs
E	Outbreaks in developing countries Particularly serious for pregnant women	Contaminated food or water

and *is* costly, because recovery may take months, it is rarely fatal. The real worry is that it could turn into "chronic hepatitis." Chronic hepatitis happens when the body doesn't entirely clear the virus. Although your symptoms may partially or completely resolve, the virus continues to multiply in your liver. After years of chronic hepatitis, a ruinous amount of scar tissue can form in the liver (cirrhosis) and/or liver cancer (hepatoma) may develop. Furthermore, you remain contagious and are somewhat of a pariah to those you contact. Chronic hepatitis sometimes heals on its own, but you cannot count on that. Medical treatments for it are toxic, expensive, and don't work very well. Clearly, hepatitis is best avoided altogether, rather than dealt with later.

So far, medical science has distinguished five different kinds of viral infections that cause hepatitis. The names are not difficult to recall: hepatitis A, B, C, D, and E. Although all of them

TABLE 11.2
Rules for preventing hepatitis

1. Before you travel to developing countries, take hepatitis A vaccine, unless you've previously had hepatitis A.

2. When traveling, eat only cooked or freshly peeled foods and drink only carbonated or boiled beverages (see table 7.1).

3. If you are exposed to hepatitis A, haven't had the disease before, and have not been vaccinated for it, you should receive a dose of gamma globulin within 72 hours.

4. Never have unprotected sex with strangers or use illicit drugs.

5. If you are at all at risk for hepatitis B, get vaccinated.

6. If you are exposed to hepatitis B and haven't had it before, you may need vaccine and/or globulin within two weeks of being exposed.

can provoke similar sets of symptoms, each one is unique. In the following sections I will point out the unique features of each of the five infections. Their salient features are also shown in table 11.1. Each type of hepatitis also requires its own separate preventive strategy which I will detail, but a comprehensive set of rules for avoiding hepatitis is set out for you in table 11.2.

Avoiding hepatitis A

Hepatitis A is the most common of the five infections. In fact one-fourth of the persons living in the United States have had it by age twenty-five and half by age forty, although many do not realize it. Fortunately, it is also the least serious; it is rarely fatal and never leads to chronic hepatitis. It can, however, make you ill for three months or more, and the care of hepatitis A costs the United States $220 million a year.

You catch hepatitis A by ingesting the virus. You swallow something the virus is on and it gets to your liver via your gut. What you ingest was contaminated by another human being's waste. (Human hepatitis viruses are not carried in other animals or on objects for very long.) The person from whom you acquired the virus is also infected, but may not become ill for up to two weeks and may be unaware they are contagious. You may or may not have direct contact with that person. It is only necessary to contact microscopic amounts of their feces.

You are most likely to contract hepatitis A in this way from two sources: (1) contaminated food and water, or (2) contact with children enrolled in day-care facilities. In either case, if you know you've been exposed, a very safe injection (immune serum globulin) will prevent the illness, provided you seek medical attention soon enough.

Some foods are especially likely to be contaminated. Shell-fish—especially oysters—are high on the list. They are filter feeders. As they siphon large amounts of water, their filters catch small bits of suspended nutrients. Inevitably, the shellfish are also concentrating all kinds of particulate matter from the water. If sewage contaminated with hepatitis A virus gets in the ocean bed where they grow, they may also be concentrating viral particles. Although shellfish are usually quite safe, it is not possible to tell which are contaminated and which are clean. I don't recommend eating raw shellfish, especially raw oysters.

Any food can carry hepatitis A if the person preparing it is shedding the virus. This is unusual in the United States, and common in the developing world (also see chapter 7). You have no way of knowing you were exposed until after the cook becomes ill, and then only if he or she is properly diagnosed and if you then are located and informed. If the food preparer is family or a friend, you are much more likely to find out that you are at risk. If you do find out you were exposed to hepatitis, it is probably not too late to do something about it.

Hepatitis A takes about a month to cause disease, and up to two weeks after you've been exposed, you can get a shot and be protected. More good news: the injection is associated with no major side effects. Although it is a human product, it has never transmitted an infection, only prevented them. It is technically called "immune serum globulin, human" and commonly called "gamma globulin." Furthermore, it works quite well, about 80 percent of the time. Although hepatitis A is quite contagious, only certain exposures warrant this injection. Get a shot of immune serum globulin if someone with hepatitis A has lived in the same household with you, has been a sexual contact of yours, or has prepared food for you in the preceding two weeks. Interpret "household" to include bunk mates, dorm mates, and children's playmates at day care.

If you expect that it will be likely that you will be exposed to hepatitis A, a new vaccine is available so that you can protect yourself. This vaccine, "hepatitis A vaccine, inactivated (Havrix)," is quite safe and effective and should soon make hepatitis A a rare thing. It was first tested on a group of children in rural New York who predictably experience an outbreak of hepatitis A each year when an influx of city kids come up for summer break. When the experimental vaccine was given to five hundred children, none developed hepatitis. The only kids who developed the disease were those who received only dummy injections. Later, it was tested on thousands of children in Thailand where it also worked quite well and gave no more side effects than a mildly sore arm. It is really quite a breakthrough.

Hepatitis A vaccine is given as a single injection. However, if your potential exposure to hepatitis A will be an ongoing problem, get a booster shot after six to eighteen months. Although it is not known how long protection from the new vaccine will last, with a booster injection, at least twenty years is likely. If you are over forty, you are likely to be immune to hepatitis A from natural infection. In that case, you may want to have a blood test for hepatitis A antibodies before receiving the vaccine. If you already have antibodies, the vaccine is unnecessary. If you forgo the blood test and are vaccinated but don't really need to be, it won't hurt you.

Hepatitis A vaccine becomes effective after two weeks. So, if you are traveling, get it at least two weeks before departure. And if you have been exposed to hepatitis A, you may want to receive the vaccine, but it may not work quickly enough. In that case, you still want to receive immune serum globulin, which can be given simultaneously with the vaccine at a different site.

How will you know you might be at risk of contacting hepatitis A and should take the hepatitis A vaccine? First, if you will be visiting a country whose food and water supply are suspect, protect yourself beforehand. The list of countries relatively safe from hepatitis A is quite short: the United States, Canada, Australia, New Zealand, and the countries of Western Europe. For travel to all other countries, you may be at risk for hepatitis A. Native Americans (including Inuits) are also at a substantial risk for hepatitis A because epidemics of it occur in their communities periodically. Persons who work at childcare centers are prone to contact hepatitis A, and parents of children in day care are at some risk as well. Lastly, if you are a food handler, avail yourself of hepatitis A vaccine, not for your own sake but for those you are serving.

Avoiding hepatitis B

Hepatitis A is a bother, but hepatitis B is serious. Unlike hepatitis A, acute hepatitis B can be fatal; about one in a hundred people who contract hepatitis B will die. And another ten may find themselves with chronic hepatitis. Even though we've had a safe and effective vaccine to prevent hepatitis B since 1982, the incidence of this disease has increased! This should not be.

Hepatitis B virus is carried in all the bodily secretions, but it is most concentrated in blood. It is usually spread by exposure to blood—and even minute amounts of contaminated blood are sufficient to bring about infection. It is only contracted from other persons. The usual ways this happens are during sex, with exposure to blood or blood products, from infected mothers to their children during childbirth, and among children during play. The average lifetime risk of contracting hepatitis B in the United States has been about 5 percent, but certain behaviors greatly increase that risk.

Sexual promiscuity definitely puts a person at high risk for hepatitis B. Although unprotected sexual intercourse probably presents the highest risk, sexual contact of other kinds can also spread the virus. And you cannot really tell from physical appearance or background who is and who is not contagious for hepatitis B, although Asians, Africans, and people who have used intravenous drugs are much more likely to carry it. Among children, ordinary play and contact sports can transmit this virus, probably through tiny scratches and cuts. Anyone who is regularly exposed to other people's blood is at high risk of carrying the virus—for example, people who work in hospitals, morticians, and drug users who share hypodermic needles. Blood transfusions have been free of hepatitis B for well over a decade.

Excellent protection from hepatitis B can be achieved with hepatitis B vaccine. Unfortunately, relatively few people have availed themselves of this protection. The only group that has commonly made use of the vaccine since it became available in 1982 has been health care workers. Many of them were required to do so as a condition of work. Why haven't other people taken advantage of the availability of the vaccine? Some may have feared that the vaccine itself was unsafe because it was derived from human plasma. That should not be a reason to turn it down: now hepatitis vaccines are genetically engineered and grown in yeast cells. They are quite safe. In fact, usually the only side effect is a bit of a sore arm.

In 1992, the American Academy of Pediatrics recommended

that *all* children receive this vaccine—both to prevent hepatitis B and to prevent cirrhosis and liver cancer much later in life. Make sure your kids get this protection. All adults who are at risk for hepatitis B should seek vaccination as well. These persons fall into two groups: those who come into contact with the blood of others, and those who are likely to contact persons carrying hepatitis B. See table 11.3 for details.

When you receive hepatitis B vaccine, be sure it is administered correctly. It must be given in a series of three doses, the second one month and the third six months after beginning. To be effective, it has to be given in the arm to adults and the front of the thigh in children, not in the buttock. It also must be given in the muscle (intramuscular), not just under the skin (intradermal). For people with weakened immune systems (for example, persons on hemodialysis or persons with HIV), each dose should be double the standard (2 cc instead of 1 cc).

Not everyone responds to this vaccine; one person in twenty doesn't get the desired response. If you want to know if you were a responder you can have a blood test to see if you have developed antibodies to the virus. It is not clear yet if or when boosters might be needed. So far the vaccine seems to last at least seven years. After that, check with your doctor for an updated recommendation.

If you know or suspect that you've been exposed, there's an excellent chance that the disease can be prevented before the virus becomes established in you. And you have some time. It takes two to three months on average to develop the disease after being exposed to hepatitis B virus, but starting treatment within two weeks after an exposure works. You should be given not only the first of three vaccine injections, but also a one-time dose of a special gamma globulin with high hepatitis B activity (hepatitis B immune globulin, or HBIG). This globulin protects you immediately, before the vaccine has had a chance to work. It is one thousand times more potent for this virus

TABLE 11.3
Adults who should receive hepatitis B vaccine

Persons likely to contact blood or blood products:
  medical workers
  morticians
  intravenous drug abusers
  persons on hemodialysis
  hemophiliacs

Persons likely to be exposed to others with hepatitis B:
  persons whose sexual partners are infected with hepatitis B
  persons with multiple sexual partners
  homosexual males
  infants of mothers who carry hepatitis B
  police officers
  prisoners and prison staff
  persons in institutions for the mentally retarded and their staff

than the ordinary gamma globulin used for hepatitis A. Receiving both HBIG and vaccine is important.

If you've received the hepatitis B vaccine in the past, and then have a known exposure to the virus (usually from a needle-stick or sex), here's what you need to do. Have your blood tested for antibodies. The usual test is "hepatitis B surface antibody" (also designated HbsAb or anti-Hbs). If it is positive (more than 10 milli-International Units per milliliter), indicating adequate immunity, you need no treatment. If the blood test is negative, your immune status is unclear. Although you may actually have some immunity left, play it safe and get one dose of HBIG in the buttock and a booster dose of the vaccine in the arm.

If you are pregnant, stopping the transfer of hepatitis to the newborn is critical. Whereas only one in ten infected adults does not clear hepatitis B virus from their liver and become a chronic carrier of the virus, nine out of ten infants exposed to it end up that way. This is why viral-induced cirrhosis and liver cancer are much more common in Asia and Africa than here. Children are not uncommonly infected at birth in developing countries, and by the time they reach young adulthood, decades of injury has already occurred and problems arise. To stop transmission to infants, pregnant women must get tested. The test to request is the hepatitis B surface antigen (also designated HbsAg). This test measures the presence of the actual virus or its protein, and identifies those who are infectious. If this is positive, warn the pediatrician to give both hepatitis B immune globulin (HBIG) and vaccine at birth. If this is done, the baby will be all right.

Avoiding hepatitis C

A lot is still unknown about hepatitis C. The virus for it was only discovered in 1988. Before then the illness was called non-A, non-B hepatitis. Fairly reliable tests for the virus only became available in 1993. Hepatitis C is a matter of concern because a high percentage of people exposed to the virus become chronic carriers—50 percent, compared to 10 percent for hepatitis B. The carriers may develop cirrhosis long after their original exposure to hepatitis C virus.

Fortunately, hepatitis C is harder to catch than other kinds of hepatitis viruses. Some of the modes of infection that make hepatitis A and B so much of a problem—infection by mouth, sexually, and from mother to child—all appear to occur rarely with hepatitis C. Hepatitis C virus is usually transmitted by blood, contaminated needles, and substance abuse.

To avoid hepatitis C, accept blood transfusions and other blood products only if absolutely necessary. Blood banks have made great strides in diminishing the risk of hepatitis C. Now only three in ten thousand blood units transmit it. Once, two antibody preparations (Gammagard and Polygam) were discovered to be contaminated with hepatitis C and to have accounted for at least 112 cases of the disease. These products were withdrawn in February 1994.

Another way you might be exposed to hepatitis C is if you were to sustain a needlestick with contaminated blood. In the past, 2 cc of immune serum globulin were given after such exposures. However, since 1992, blood donors (from whom the globulin is harvested) have been tested for hepatits C and are excluded if antibodies to it are found. Therefore, the product no longer contains antibodies to hepatitis C and is of no value in this setting. There is no vaccine for hepatitis C yet.

Avoiding hepatitis D

Hepatitis D (or delta) is a serious but rare and unusual infection. It is unique in that it will only infect persons with a preceding or concomitant hepatitis B infection. If you avoid hepatitis B (see above), you will never get delta hepatitis. If you are chronically infected with hepatitis B, you are susceptible. Worse, whereas being infected with both viruses at the same time usually clears up, getting hepatitis D after getting type B leads to chronic hepatitis 90 percent of the time, usually leading to cirrhosis. Hepatitis D generally occurs in drug users who share needles. If you use intravenous drugs you will want to read chapter 12 carefully, as well.

Avoiding hepatitis E

Hepatitis E is transmitted like hepatitis A: the virus has to enter your body through your mouth. The disease has not been found in the United States or Canada. It is common in Asia, especially India, and in Africa. In North America it has only been found in rural Mexico. In these countries it causes large epidemics. Hepatitis E may be fatal about 1 percent of the time. Pregnant women are particularly at risk; almost 15 percent of them may die. There is no vaccine for hepatitis E, but if you follow the cardinal rules given in chapter 7 for eating abroad you should not be at risk.

12 *HIV infection and AIDS*

*T*he acquired immune deficiency syndrome (AIDS) is a fatal viral infection caused by the human immune deficiency virus (HIV). When people contract this virus, they are said to be "HIV-positive" from then on. Although they might not show any sign of illness for a long time, the virus is silently and seriously injuring their immune system. When their immune defenses are critically weakened, they develop AIDS. At this point, organisms we commonly contact and easily ward off can cause serious and ultimately fatal infections.

HIV can cause countless different medical problems, but a typical course of the infection goes something like this (see table 12.1): Only a few weeks after contracting HIV, half the infected persons will have a transient illness similar to infectious mononucleosis, often including fever, headache, swollen glands, and rash. Then, for years, most HIV-infected persons will have no symptoms. Nevertheless, during this time the virus is slowly destroying immune cells in the lymph nodes. Because the virus is also circulating in the bloodstream, these apparently healthy persons can pass the virus to other people. After about eight years on the average, the immune system is substantially maimed and a series of new infections occur. Most of these infections are more or less unique to persons with AIDS and are treatable. (They will be discussed in detail in chapter 14 because there are ways people with HIV can avoid many of them.) However, eventually, untreatable infections (or cancers) develop, and patients weaken, lose weight, and may suffer

TABLE 12.1
Estimated number of individuals newly infected with HIV

North America	36,000–54,000
Caribbean	45,000–80,000
Latin America	120,000–180,000
Western Europe	30,000–40,000
North Africa & Middle East	43,000–67,000
Sub-Saharan Africa	3.0–3.4 million
Eastern Europe & Central Asia	180,000–280,000
East Asia & Pacific	150,000–270,000
South & Southeast Asia	610,000–1.1 million
Australia & New Zealand	700–1,000
Total:	**4.2–5.8 million**

SOURCE: World Health Organization, 2003.

chronic diarrhea, visual loss, or mental deterioration before death occurs.

AIDS deserves its infamy. Approximately one million people in the United States are living with HIV. Even if no one else contracted the virus, these million Americans will remain contagious for HIV. Already, HIV infects forty thousand people a year in the United States alone, where it is the major cause of death in young men and is a rapidly increasing cause of death in young women. Internationally, the new infection rate is much higher (see figure 12.1).

HIV is nearly always contracted through sex, from contaminated needles and blood, and by fetuses from their mothers. These three modes of transmission are so predominant that all other modes of transmission are eclipsed in importance. Nevertheless, rarer ways of getting AIDS are equally fatal, equally terrifying, and equally preventable, so I will discuss them as well.

Contracting HIV through sex

Sexual intercourse with a person infected with HIV is the most common way AIDS is transmitted. The only way you can be certain to avoid sexually transmitted HIV infection is to avoid sex with any partner who might carry the virus. There are only two ways to be confident that a person is HIV-negative: First, if an American has engaged in no high-risk behavior since HIV started here in 1979, they can be presumed to be HIV-negative. Otherwise, only a negative HIV blood test can be trusted. Because it can take six months after infection before the blood test "converts"—that is, shows evidence of infection—you must feel confident the blood was drawn six months or more following their last risky behavior.

Remember, there are no physical characteristics that you can rely on to identify a person who might transmit HIV. In my practice, I have cared for HIV-infected executives, homemakers, soldiers, and grandparents. Make no assumptions about someone's potential communicability based on their appearance or their background.

Having sex with persons whose HIV status is unknown is unsafe, but I recognize that (a) it is often difficult to be sure about someone's HIV status, and (b) many are willing to undertake some element of risk when it comes to sexual encounters. The only other method currently available to substantially diminish—but not eliminate—the risk of HIV transmitted by sex is proper use of the male latex condom. In studies performed in Europe, when heterosexual couples consistently used condoms correctly, and one was HIV-positive and the other was HIV-negative, the uninfected partner always remained uninfected. When similar couples were not consistent in their use of condoms, HIV was transmitted at a rate of 12.7 percent over a two-year period of exposure. It passed equally well from man to woman as from woman to man.

No other method has proven as good at preventing the

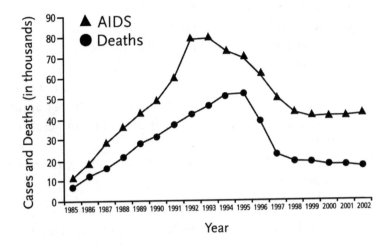

FIGURE 12.1 *AIDS and AIDS deaths in the United States, 1985–2005*
The death rate from AIDS rose rapidly until 1996.
SOURCE: Centers for Disease Control and Prevention.

sexual transmission of HIV. Do not expect male condoms made of other materials, contraceptive sponges, nonoxynol-9 (spermicidal jelly), or coitus interruptus ("pulling out") to protect you or your partner if one of you is infected with HIV. Also, although HIV passes more easily in certain circumstances—if there are genital sores and rashes, if anal intercourse is practiced, or during menses—none of these conditions is necessary for the virus to be transmitted.

If you are going to depend on a condom for protection from HIV, you must use it properly. Here are some essential guidelines to follow, or to insist that your male partner follow, if the condom is to be reliable:

1. Be sure the container and wrapping are undamaged.
2. Apply the condom after the penis is erect, but piror to any genital contact.

3. Leave a small airspace at the tip if one is not built in; this will allow room for the ejaculate.
4. Roll the condom all the way to the base of the penis.
5. Ensure adequate lubrication. If this doesn't happen naturally, use a water-based lubricant such as K-Y Jelly.
6. Never allow an oil-based lubricant to contact the condom; these can dissolve latex. Therefore, do not apply massage oils, vegetable oils or shortening, mineral oil, or petroleum jelly.
7. Hold the condom to the base of the penis on withdrawal to avoid spillage.
8. Use a new condom with each sexual act.

Recently, a female condom (Reality) has been marketed. Its ability to prevent transmission of HIV is unknown. Therefore, don't depend on it for this purpose. In fact, Reality is reported to have a failure rate of 11 percent in preventing pregnancy, so it clearly does not always provide a complete barrier.

What we know about the risk of sexual intercourse is still unknown for other sexual acts. Not enough is known, for example, about deep kissing and orogenital sex. Since HIV has been found in saliva, semen, and cervical secretions (although in much lower concentrations than in blood), and since various common sores of the mouth and gums can bleed from time to time, these activities do carry some risk of their own. Indeed, we know that penetration by a penis is not required. There have now been five well-documented cases of transmission of HIV by female homosexual activity. It is best to refrain from deep kissing and orogenital sex unless you know your partner is HIV-negative.

Contracting HIV from hypodermic needles

The second major means of transmitting HIV (and therefore AIDS) is through contaminated needles—that is, needles contaminated with blood infected with the virus. By and large, the risk here is the hollow-bore needle, the type used to inject drugs and medicines. It is interesting that no surgeon has yet contracted HIV at work. During accidents and operations, scalpels, knives, razors, and the like usually don't carry enough blood on them to transmit the infection. But the hollow bore needle is a tube, and, although it is quite slender, a sufficient volume of blood can be carried there and deposited under the skin of another person.

The vast majority of people with HIV and AIDS who have contracted the disease through needles are users of cocaine, heroin, and other addictive substances that are taken by injection. Should you fall into this category, you should be aware that the drugs affect your ability to think clearly and thus to take precautions consistently. So I urge you to seek help in breaking the drug habit (it can't be done alone) as well as to follow precautions against contracting HIV. Recognizing that addiction is extremely difficult to break, I offer the following guidelines (adapted from the U.S. Public Health Service's Center for Substance Abuse Treatment) for those who continue:

1. Never share needles. Remember, you cannot tell by people's appearance, character, or background whether they might be infected with HIV.
2. Use a needle only once and then discard it in a pierce-proof closed container.
3. Use only sterile needles from unopened, undamaged containers. If there is a needle exchange program in your state, take advantage of it.
4. If you must reuse needles, sterilize them as follows: Take the plunger, syringe, and needle apart and rinse off all visible blood. Then, soak in undiluted household bleach for at least thirty seconds. Put the equipment back together and flush with bleach three times. Then, rinse

the needle and syringe by filling at least three times with fresh, preferably sterile (boiled), water. In each step, fill the syringe to the very top. Shaking and tapping the syringe during the process will also improve its effectiveness. Cleaning both before and after use is best.

There are situations other than illicit drug use in which HIV can be passed by needle injection. These include transfusion of contaminated blood products and occupational needlestick accidents.

Transfusion of blood and blood products is, overall, the third most common way persons in the United States have contracted HIV infection. Fortunately, this is now extremely uncommon. Since April 1985 all donated blood has been tested for antibodies to HIV. This step, when added to questioning donors and excluding those with any personal risk factors, has decreased the risk of acquiring HIV from a single unit of blood or plasma to far less than one in one hundred thousand. Nevertheless, HIV has not been—and may never be—totally eliminated from blood transfusions. Donors may either lie or be ignorant about risks. They may have been infected very recently, and the tests for HIV may not yet be able to detect the infection. And there always exists some chance of test failure and/or clerical error.

What can an individual do to further minimize the risk of contracting HIV from a blood transfusion? First, although physicians are more hesitant than ever to order transfusions, it is still wise for patient or family to respectfully discuss the need for a particular transfusion, especially if the patient is not actively bleeding. (Ask: "Would it be safe to wait and see what the blood count is tomorrow?" "Would iron or vitamins help reverse this anemia?")

If you have elective surgery planned, store blood. Generally, you can bank up to four units of your own blood within six weeks of surgery. However, asking relatives or friends to donate, called "directed donation," may not be the best idea. Directed donations may be a higher risk than random blood bank blood. Whereas most donors are anonymous and have no reason to answer the blood bank's questions untruthfully, relatives may not be willing to admit high-risk behavior. They might not want to explain to the family later why they were rejected as donors (or why they should have been). You can also have your own blood frozen for up to ten years, but this blood is not as good as fresh blood and it may be logistically hard to get if you need it in an emergency. The high cost of maintaining frozen blood may not be worth it.

Persons with hemophilia have a special need for blood products. When faced with bleeding, the factor they lack (factor VIII) must be given as "antihemophilic factor" or AHF. None of the available AHFs are now infected with HIV. Some are still made from human blood, but sterilization techniques seem to have been perfected. Unfortunately, though, most persons who were treated before 1985 for hemophilia are already infected with HIV transmitted through blood products.

Finally, HIV has been spread by means of needles in the workplace. Considering the great number of exposures medical workers have had to the blood of HIV-positive individuals in the United States since this epidemic began, work-related transmission is extremely uncommon. Hospital workers have contracted HIV most often when hollow-bore needles contaminated with HIV-positive blood accidentally pierced their skin. As you might expect, the affected personnel have predominantly been nurses and blood-drawers. Although rare—less than a hundred cases are known to have been contracted by this means—these are tragic occurrences.

If all hospital guidelines were followed, transmission in this manner would be minimal. Hospital workers are now required to attend classes on "universal precautions." These are guidelines that, if learned and followed, should eliminate nearly all dangerous exposures in the medical workplace. The term "universal" refers to the fact that in the hospital *all* blood and body fluids, regardless of source, are now handled as if they were contaminated. Since hospital care workers should be well versed on prevention techniques, I will offer just one piece of simple advice that can reduce medical personnel's risk to near zero. When you must handle a needle, never allow any part of your body, especially your free hand, to be forward of the needle tip. Never aim a needle at yourself, or, for that matter, in the direction of others. The same rule should be followed for any instrument sharp enough to penetrate skin. This rule would forbid the recapping of needles and a range of other unwise maneuvers. The only needlestick injuries that could still occur would be freak accidents.

If you are stuck by a needle, what can you do? First, don't overreact. If the needle merely scratched or brushed your skin and there is no visible blood drawn from your person, the exposure is not significant. If there is no visible blood on the needle, in the syringe, or on the sharp object, you are not in danger. However, if there is a skin-penetrating injury with a bloody object, immediately clean the wound. Use the handiest disinfectant; bleach, Betadine, alcohol, and most other disinfectants kill HIV well. Get the disinfectant as deep into the wound as you can, but injection, surgery, or amputation is not indicated. After that, consider starting medication.

If you feel sure the blood contained HIV, consider starting AZT (Retrovir) along with one or two other anti-HIV medicines. The exact regimen depends on the source and degree of your exposure and is a choice taken with your doctor's advice. However, if you are going to do so, start immediately; experiments in animals show that if it is going to help it must be started shortly after injury. The medicines are continued for one month.

They will not always work, but they are widely thought to be of potential benefit.

Lastly, try to find out if the blood to which you were exposed was indeed infected. Either have the blood of the "donor" tested or have the object tested; this can be done even after the blood has dried. If the blood is HIV-negative, stop AZT, of course, and breathe a sigh of relief. If you were inoculated with HIV-positive blood, you chances of becoming infected are still quite low: only one chance in two hundred.

To monitor your own blood, have HIV tests on the day of injury, six weeks later, and again six months later. The few persons who pick up HIV through accidental needlesticks will generally have a positive blood test at six weeks; rarely, it takes six months to convert, but never longer.

Passing HIV from mother to infant

Transmission of HIV from mother to newborn child is yet another common way the disease is spread. This completes a triad that accounts for the overwhelming majority of cases: sex, needles, and childbearing. Because the baby has no way to protect itself, it is up to the mother to prevent the child from contracting the virus. There are several things she can do.

HIV can pass from mother to child during pregnancy, delivery, and infancy. At the time you find out you are pregnant, you need to have an HIV blood test. If it is negative, it is imperative that you follow all the guidelines in this chapter to keep yourself and the fetus from being infected. A fetus or newborn baby can only become infected with HIV if its mother is infected first. (An infected father does not spread HIV directly to a future infant at the time of conception.) Furthermore, when you are newly infected, the amount of virus circulating in your blood is quite high, so risk of transmission is also very high.

If you are pregnant and your test for HIV is positive, there is a substantial risk—30 percent—that the fetus will become infected. The reason that 70 percent of fetuses with HIV-positive mothers are not born HIV-positive is that maternal and fetal blood are not supposed to mix. They are separated in the placenta by narrow membranes. Breaks in the membranes are not uncommon, though, and that is why many children of HIV-infected mothers also have the virus at the time of birth.

Treatment for these mothers and their infants markedly improves the children's chances of escaping infection. Infants of mothers who did not receive the drug AZT were infected 25.5 percent of the time. But in a similar group that received AZT, only 8.3 percent of the babies had contracted the virus. The treatment is fairly complex: the mother starts AZT during the fourteenth week of pregnancy. Data from a registry of women who have taken AZT during pregnancy indicate that these women's fetuses do not have an increased risk of malformation. During labor, AZT is given intravenously. After delivery, AZT syrup is given to the infant for six weeks. If the mother takes *three* HIV drugs, the infection rate is even lower.

The choice to request an abortion is a difficult one. Moral convictions play a primary role. The chance that the baby may get AIDS also enters into the decision. Two other aspects of HIV and childbirth should also be considered: the risk of becoming ill during pregnancy, and the prospect that the child might ultimately become orphaned.

Pregnancy itself is an immune-suppressing condition. The number of lymphocytes—cells that specialize in fighting infection-causing viruses and bacteria—normally drops in pregnancy. The lymphocyte count drops even more quickly during pregnancy in women who are HIV-positive. Pregnant women are ordinarily at special risk from infections such as chickenpox and urinary tract infections, and infections are more common and more serious for pregnant women who are HIV-positive. If the father is also HIV-positive—as is usually the case—the chance the baby ultimately will be orphaned is to be considered, although if HIV-positive parents take all their medicines and keep their viral load low, they may lead a normal life.

Newborns not uncommonly become infected during the act of delivery, as well. Does the method of delivery matter? Recently, Dr. Louise Kuhn of Columbia University in New York City showed that the way the baby is delivered can matter, at least in complicated cases. Infants delivered by uncomplicated cesarean section (C-section) procedures were infected with HIV roughly half as often as those with complicated vaginal deliveries: those with prolonged labor, those requiring manipulation of the baby's position, those with bleeding, and so on. The difference between the infection rate of babies born by C-section and those with normal, uncomplicated vaginal delivery was much less significant. Other precautions obstetricians should take include avoiding amniocentesis (sampling the fluid in the womb by needle) or using the protruding baby's scalp for monitoring, as with electrodes.

At delivery, testing can determine if the baby is already infected with HIV. Request the PCR test (PCR stands for polymerase chain reaction), which can identify the virus in the baby's blood. The routine tests for HIV are confused by the mother's antibodies, which cross the placenta. If the baby escaped infection during pregnancy, do not breast-feed. Breast milk, especially shortly after delivery, may contain large amounts of HIV, and infants can become infected by ingesting it.

Rare modes of transmission

We have discussed so far how not to transmit HIV by means of sex, hypodermic needles (drug abuse, transfusions, and accidents), and from mother to child. That covers over 99 percent of what you need to know to protect yourself from AIDS, because over 99 percent of people with HIV were infected in one of these three ways. However, there is great concern about other possible ways to get AIDS. If you follow every precaution I've advised thus far, are you totally safe?

It has been widely publicized that six persons contracted HIV by visiting a dentist. This all happened in only one dental practice, and there are no reports of it happening again. This outbreak also occurred before the start of new and specific sterilization and infection control guidelines for dentists. You may want to ask if your dentist follows the CDC guidelines. If so, your risk is minuscule. In fact, several studies have focused on dentists who were identified as HIV-positive. The researchers looked back at the patients these dentists had treated. In none of these studies were any patients found who had contracted HIV at the dentist's office. The most careful of these studies (by Dr. Jenice Longfield) looked at 2,753 patients treated by a pediatric dentist after he had become infected with HIV. He performed oral surgery on 20 percent of them, and none of his patients contracted HIV.

No cases of HIV transmission have been attributed to procedures performed by an HIV-infected surgeon. At least four look-back studies have been done searching for such patients. No, you would not necessarily be informed if your surgeon—or, for that matter, other operating room (OR) personnel—were HIV-positive. In any case, surgeons and OR nurses are just as concerned as you are about the integrity of OR barriers between patient and doctor. Breaks in technique (for example, gloves ripped on bone chips) do occur with some regularity in the surgical arena. However, the fact is that these exposures have not been sufficient to spread HIV. To look at it in another way, there have been myriad surgical procedures done on HIV-infected patients since AIDS came to this country, especially in the trauma centers of New York, San Francisco, and Miami. Yet, not one surgeon has been infected from his or her patients. Of the many concerns that accompany surgery (see chapter 16), HIV is a relatively trivial one.

Blood spills can occur in the hospital setting, but also in sports and at the scene of an accident. It is best, of course, not to touch blood with bare hands. If gloves are not available, cover your hands with a plastic bag or other material. However, HIV cannot penetrate intact skin. In the extremely rare instances in which HIV has been transmitted after blood spills, transmission occurred to someone with a rash, sore, or open wound on their uncovered hands. The most convenient way to clean up and sterilize a blood spill is to cleanse the area with household bleach. A mixture of one part bleach to one hundred parts water (one quarter cup bleach in one gallon tap water) is sufficient.

Rarely, transmission can occur at home through intimate contact with the blood and/or body secretions (saliva, urine, and stool) of an infected person. Only eight cases like this are known to have occurred, and they happened as follows:

1. A mother acquired HIV after caring for an HIV-infected child. The mother's tasks included drawing the child's blood, giving him intravenous therapy, and cleaning up his stool, but she did not wear gloves.
2. A mother injected blood factors for each of two hemophiliac sons, only one of whom was HIV-positive. She used less than optimal technique and the uninfected brother picked up the virus.
3. A child with a heavily scratched rash became infected with HIV while living in the same household with another HIV-positive child who suffered from frequent bleeding.
4. HIV passed from one adolescent to another; they both had hemophilia, shared razors, and cut themselves while shaving.

5. An HIV-positive person bit another household member who later also tested positive for HIV.

6. A child converted to HIV-positive while living with two parents dying of AIDS. The child's mother had extensive skin rashes that often bled. The child had impetigo and abrasions herself, and her mother cared for these barehanded. The child frequently hugged and slept with the mother, and sometimes used the father's toothbrush.

7. The caretaker of an AIDS patient became infected with the virus. She had rashes and small cuts on her hands, but did not wear gloves when tending to the patient.

8. An elderly mother provided extensive home nursing for her son as he was dying of AIDS. He had intermittent bleeding from the gums and the bowels. She inconsistently wore gloves and became HIV-positive as well.

From these examples, you can see that HIV can spread in the household when proper precautions are bypassed. If you are caring for or living with an HIV-positive person, take utmost care with needles. Be sure you are thoroughly educated in their safe use before accepting the task. If possible, use occlusive bandages to cover all breaks in the skin, both your own wounds and those on the HIV-positive person. Wear disposable gloves whenever there is the possibility of contacting blood or bodily secretions. Take care when cleaning spills of blood and bodily secretions, as previously advised. Wash your hands with a germicidal soap after contact with such fluids, even if you had been wearing gloves.

Caring for an AIDS patient is very safe, as long as you are careful. Further information on this topic is available in the CDC's pamphlet *Caring for Someone with AIDS*. Call (800) 458-5231 to request a free copy.

How you will _not_ get AIDS

HIV is transmitted by intimate contact with an HIV-infected individual, but it is *not* transmitted by casual contact. It is not transmitted by merely touching HIV-positive people, by sharing a glass, or by sharing a bathroom with them. How is this known? First, almost everyone who has contracted AIDS in this country has fallen into one of the major risk groups. In over two decades of treating HIV infection myself, no patients I've cared for have developed AIDS without first having been exposed sexually, by intravenous drug use, or by transfusion. Patients are not stricken with AIDS out of the blue.

Second, there have been over fourteen combined prospective surveys of over 750 individuals exposed to HIV in the household, and not a single case of HIV infection was identified. Although I have told you that household transmission can happen, these surveys show that it is extremely rare; HIV-positive persons do not transmit the virus just by living together with others. Similarly, there is no evidence that HIV has been transmitted in the school setting. HIV-positive children should not be barred from attending school, and their classmates should not be concerned about picking up HIV during classroom activities.

AIDS is not transmitted by insects. Early in the U.S. epidemic, epidemiologists were concerned about the potential for transmission by mosquitoes or flies. The pattern of transmission never fit this hypothesis in any case. Nevertheless, when investigators led by Dr. Patricia Webb took it one step further and tried their best to infect mosquitos and biting flies, they could not do so, even under optimal laboratory conditions. Furthermore, they measured the volume of blood the insects could carry in their mouth and demonstrated that the amount was inadequate to transmit HIV.

There is no evidence that HIV can be spread through the

air; in spas, swimming pools, and saunas; or on exercise equipment or other inanimate objects. It is not contracted by having blood drawn or by donating blood. And it is not transmitted by a handshake or a hug, two things that those unfortunate enough to be infected with this dreaded virus appreciate enormously.

Four

Persons with unique risks

13　*Special persons and special situations*

There are many reasons your immune system may not be up to par from time to time. If you recently had a viral infection or your nutrition has been poor, your immune system can't fight germs as well as usual. However, certain specific and severe immune problems can be permanent, and AIDS is not the only one. When you have one of these other problems, for example diabetes or kidney disease, you have a unique type of immune weakness. You become susceptible for a particular set of infections, different for each disease. Many are preventable, if you are forewarned. First, however, there are certain general things you can do to shore up your defenses if for any reason your immune system is not working normally.

Cutting fats to prevent heart disease, cutting calories to lose weight, and fine tuning your carbohydrates to control diabetes are among the many good reasons to adjust your diet. But your immune system works with proteins. And vitamins are needed for the proteins to function. So if you do not have an adequate protein and vitamin intake, your immune system does not have the building blocks it requires to fight off germs. (An extreme example: the pneumonia that is now mostly found in people with AIDS was first noted in starving children after World War II.) For each kilogram you weigh, take in at least 1 gram of protein per day—about 70 grams for an average adult. If you are eating at least 1,200 calories daily, and all food groups are represented, your diet contains sufficient vitamins. Otherwise, take a multivitamin. Although taking megavitamins is a current fad, there's no proof that it benefits or restores immune function.

Get a flu shot each year around November 1 and get the pneumonia shot once (see chapter 8). Have a skin test for TB yearly and consider taking medication if it is positive (see chapter 9). Limit contact with contagious persons whenever possible. If you will be traveling abroad, review your itinerary with an infectious disease specialist or travel clinic at least a month before you depart (see chapter 7). And pay particular attention to any type of injury in which the skin is broken.

Caring for wounds

Wounds are a common conduit for germs. The single most important way to get bacteria out of a wound is to wash them out. It is best to do this with sterile solutions, but they are often not around when you need them. If this is the case, tap water is the next best choice. If you're out camping, use boiled water, treated water, filtered water, or clear running stream water, in that order of preference. The key is volume. Wash the wound out copiously. Besides washing germs out of the wound, you are flushing out any foreign material (sand, gravel, lint, and the like). Foreign material in a wound can increase its propensity to become infected by a factor of ten thousand!

After irrigating the wound, pat it dry with sterile gauze. If sterile gauze is unavailable, use something clean and dry that won't leave lint, like a previously washed handkerchief or sock. Never touch an open wound with bare hands.

After drying the wound, apply a germicide. There are several choices. Iodophor (Betadine) and triple antibiotic ointment (Neosporin) are two good choices that don't sting or burn. Lastly, cover the wound with a bandage that completely seals it off to particulate matter but allows air to enter; that is, use one that is occlusive but breathes. If a Band-Aid fits, that's just fine. If you make a gauze bandage, be sure to tape the whole perimeter or it will surely slip. Assuming you've had tetanus shots before, get a booster if you've not had one in five years. (Ten years is the usual interval if you have no deep or especially dirty wound.)

Cortisone and related medicines

The archetypical double-edged sword in medicine is a class of drugs called corticosteroids. You have probably heard of one of these, cortisone. These drugs are often used to relieve the misery of poison ivy rashes and they are often injected directly into chronically inflamed joints. They can be lifesaving, too, in diseases such as asthma and some types of kidney failure and arthritis. However, they can be life threatening as well. They can severely impair your immune function and make you unduly susceptible to a wide range of infections.

The best way to avoid the ravages of corticosteroids is not to take them. I treated one critically ill man for simultaneous Legionnaires' disease and yeast meningitis. He had been given a cortisone for mild arthritis, although an aspirin-type product might also have worked. The steroids he received were the only reason he was susceptible to these germs. Without them, he never would have come down with these two infections.

The next best way to limit the complications of cortisones is to limit their dose or duration. The most commonly used drugs in this class actually don't include cortisone anymore; prednisone and Medrol are the customary ones now. If you take more than 20 mg of these per day for more than five days, you are starting to suppress your immune defenses. The more you take and the longer you take them, the worse your immune function gets. Continuous use is worse than intermittent use. If you must take a cortisonelike agent, work with your doctor to try a dose every other day. If this works, your immune system may be spared. Corticosteroid joint injections are dosed intermittently, too, but the form of the drug usually used there is slow-released and long-acting. Don't take these any more frequently than once every other month.

If you absolutely require a corticosteroid for a long period at a high dose, there are certain other parts of this book I want you to read well. They include the sections on Legionnaires' disease and pneumonia (chapter 8), and tuberculosis (chapter 9). Also, follow the guidelines recommended for HIV-positive persons (chapter 14) to avoid yeast infection (Candida), coccidioidomycosis ("cocci"), cryptococcosis ("crypto"), and herpes simplex virus.

Diabetes

More than fourteen million people in the United States have diabetes mellitus. If you are not a diabetic yourself, you probably have a friend or family member who is. Diabetics are one group of people who can overcome their immune problems if they learn about them and take precautions. The infections that occur most frequently in diabetics are listed in table 13.1.

Diabetes puts you at increased risk for infections in large part because pus-forming, infection-fighting white blood cells function poorly when the blood glucose is over 250 mg. Anyone with diabetes knows what that means. Strive always for optimal control—blood sugars closer to 100 mg—but promise yourself that you will stay under 250. However, the most common diabetes-associated infection—infected foot ulcers—happens for other reasons.

Infected foot ulcers occur more frequently than all other diabetes-associated infections combined. Worse, they lead to amputation, which happens to 60,000 diabetics each year in the United States. Furthermore, amputation is usually avoidable.

Here's how it usually works. With diabetes, there is loss of sensation in the feet. This does take years to develop, but since many people have diabetes for years before they know it, sen-

TABLE 13.1
Infections more common in people with diabetes

Yeast infections
    Thrush (white coating on tongue or throat)
    Vulvovaginitis (cottage cheese discharge and/or red rash in women)
Urinary tract infections
Staph skin infections
    Furuncles (boils)
    Carbuncles (deep skin abscesses that need surgery)
Tuberculosis
Mucormycosis (a fungus that invades the sinuses only when diabetes is
    out of control)
Foot infections
    Infected neurotropic ulcers (skin rubbed off and then attacked by
      bacteria)
    Osteomyelitis (when the infection gets down to bone)
    Wet gangrene (when it starts to invade and destroy the tissues and
      spread up the leg)

sation might already be dulled by the time you find out you have it. You lose the delicate warning systems of touch, pain, and position. Minor injuries occur and recur. And because of repeated trauma (and the impeded blood flow that also goes along with diabetes), you tend not to heal. You have now formed the infamous diabetic foot ulcer. An ulcer is a place where the body's surface—here, the skin—is absent. The feet harbor ample bacteria, and they often grow on these ulcers. Under certain conditions they can invade the ulcer, and the infection then spreads beyond the original borders of the ulcer, up the leg. If gangrene sets in, amputation becomes necessary.

With care this scenario can be avoided. Unfortunately, I see many diabetic patients who have ignored their feet until it is too late. Perhaps this is because the problem comes on gradually, or because we don't spend much time looking at our feet, or because with poor nerve function it doesn't hurt. The point is that, if you are diabetic, you have to establish a routine for yourself to follow to ensure that you properly care for your feet. No one will do this for you.

Inspect your feet completely twice daily. Apply a moisturizing cream to any dry areas. Put powder, gauze, or lamb's wool between any two toes that are rubbing. If you find the skin itchy, peeling, or scaly between the toes, it may be athlete's foot, a fungal infection. Apply Lamisil to those areas until the infection goes away. Keep your nails trimmed, preferably by filing. A long nail can cut right into a toe without your knowing it. Calluses make it difficult to fit into shoes well. Keep calluses smoothed down with a pumice stone.

Shoes that fit well are crucial. Remember, you won't feel them rubbing you the wrong way. First, buy leather shoes, which mold to your feet better than synthetics do. They must be wide enough not to pinch your feet. When they are new, wear them no more than two hours per day. When you inspect your feet, inspect the insides of your shoes also. If you find signs of wear that indicate a point of heavy contact, see if you can get the shoes stretched or adjusted, or find a new pair.

You may also have difficulty feeling temperature properly. I've seen several diabetic patients who have burned their feet on hot pavement in the summertime. Test bath water with your hands, not your feet, and don't use heating pads or hot water bottles on your feet. Splinters and glass are serious problems for a diabetic as well. Don't go around barefooted.

Even if you've followed all these rules, you may still find a place where your skin has broken down. Do not ignore it. Consider it serious and a semiemergency. Get professional care quickly. Your doctor can clean the affected skin carefully, trim infected tissue, help you get your blood sugar under control, and prescribe antibiotics if they are needed. But the single most important way to help an ulcer to heal is to get all the pressure off it. Short of bed rest, a special shoe or cast may be needed.

Cancer

Cancer is not a single disease. The different kinds of cancer arise from different types of cells, in different organs, and go through different stages. As you might imagine, the infections people with cancer are prone to are eclectic as well, and I cannot catalog them all for you here. But the most important risk common to most cancer patients is infection after chemotherapy. Chemotherapy sets you up for infection because it does not confine itself to knocking out the cancer cells—it also destroys or weakens the bone marrow where a type of white blood cell called a neutrophil is produced. A neutrophil's job is literally to engulf and kill bacteria and yeasts. They are essential infantrymen of your immune system.

You can measure your risk of infection after chemotherapy by calculating your absolute neutrophil count, or ANC. (Sometimes the term "granulocyte" is used instead of neutrophil and it becomes the AGC.) If you look at your complete blood count (CBC), you can calculate your ANC as follows. First determine your percentage of neutrophils. Do this by adding the percentages of two types of cells: the "segs" (or "polys") and the "bands" (or "immature forms"). Multiply your percentage of neutrophils by the total white blood cell count and divide by 100 (see figure 13.1).

If your ANC is over 1,000, there is no added risk of infection. Between 500 and 1,000, infections you might have gotten anyway are more likely to become serious. But below 500, the bacteria already inside your bowels, respiratory tract, or on your skin have an opportunity to invade your system and cause serious damage. An absolute neutrophil count below 100 is called "profound neutropenia," and an infection is virtually certain.

There are a few things you can do after chemotherapy to prevent problems while you are waiting for your bone marrow to make adequate neutrophils again. When the ANC drops below 500, start this plan.

The report:

White blood cell count*	4.8×10^3
% granulocytes**	30%
% bands***	5%

The calculation:

ANC = % neutrophils × white blood cell count ÷ 100
% neutrophils = % granulocytes + % bands
% neutrophils = 30 + 5 = 35
ANC = 35 × 4,800 ÷ 100 = 420

*   The white blood cell count is often abbreviated WBC.
** The granulocytes may also be called polys, segs, polymorphonuclear cells, or segmented neutrophils.
*** The bands are often called immature neutrophils or immatures.

FIGURE 13.1 *Calculating your absolute neutrophil count*

Stay out of the hospital if you can. The vast majority of germs patients get sick from when their neutrophils are low are those already residing on or in their body. The makeup of these germs is determined by your environment, and if your environment is the hospital, you will become colonized by the germs found there. In chapter 16, I will discuss the special dangers hospital germs pose. If you must stay in the hospital, insist that anyone who touches you wash their hands or don new gloves just beforehand.

Maintain a cooked diet. The very germs that are most likely to infect you when your ANC is down—*Pseudomonas,* for example—are found on salads and fresh fruits. If the low white blood cell count persists for too long, you will become at risk for fungi in addition to bacteria, and the most worrisome of these is called *Aspergillus.* This mold enters your system through the air; you breathe it in. *Aspergillus* is especially common in buildings that are under construction or being torn down. It likes to grow in the dust and fireproofing above ceilings. When this area is disturbed, you can have an invisible rain of *Aspergillus.* Stay clear of any construction, both in or out of the hospital.

TABLE 13.2
Early signs of infection when your white blood cell count is low

Symptom or sign to immediately point out to your doctor	Possible infection it might represent
Shaking chill	Bacteria in the bloodstream
Facial pain or congestion	Sinusitis
Cough	Pneumonia
Chest pain on deep breathing	Pneumonia
Rectal pain, drainage, or lumps	Rectal abscess
Sore or crust in the nose	Aspergillosis
Red skin bumps	Yeast in the blood
Nausea, vomiting	Yeast in the liver

If your ANC is low, you should be vigilant for the earliest signs of an infection and tell your doctor immediately. In addition to promptly reporting fever and chills, there are certain more specific things to watch for, listed in table 13.2.

Your doctor may put you on certain medications to reduce the chances of infection. Several antibiotics have been shown to decrease the chance of an infection occurring during neutropenia. However, the use of antibiotics is controversial because they could lead to the survival of drug-resistant germs. The other medications that might help are called growth factors. These shots, called G-CSF (Neupogen) and GM-CSF (Leukine), can sometimes stimulate the bone marrow to start producing neutrophils earlier than it otherwise would.

Transplantation

Organ transplantation has graduated from the experimental realm into the medical mainstream. Despite the many successes in prolonging the lives and well-being of people whose livers, hearts, kidneys, or bone marrow have failed, transplantation remains a complicated ordeal. Its most prominent complication is infection. Most transplant patients get through the surgery without difficulty, and new drugs do an excellent job preventing organ rejection. This leaves infection as your number one worry if you are a transplant recipient. Here's why.

Unless your donor is your identical twin, your immune system will regard a transplanted organ as "foreign" and your white blood cells will attack it. To prevent this from happening, you must take medicines that slow your immune function. These usually include cyclosporine A (Sandimmune) and the cortisone relative, prednisone. So, in order to prevent rejection of your transplant, you are rendered less able to reject germs. And it's a fine balance: too little immune-suppressing drugs and your transplanted organ may fail; too much and, before you know it, any microbe around will be feasting on you.

Your transplant team will need to suppress your immune system drastically just after transplantation. At that point, you are in a very protected environment and watched very carefully. Later, when you leave the hospital, you must do more of the watching yourself.

Transplant patients are especially prone to a certain set of infections. These are not unique to transplant recipients but often affect them differently than other people. I'll go through the most important infections for you, often referring to other sections of this book, and pointing out some distinctions of the transplant situation.

Simply by being in the hospital for the transplant surgery you can get the same hospital-acquired infections anyone else can. (Read chapter 16 before you go.) Both transplant patients and pregnant women must worry about a bacterium called *Listeria*. The pregnant woman may have a miscarriage as a result of *Listeria* infection; the transplant patient tends to get meningitis. Nevertheless, the means of prevention are the same (see chapter 15). Legionnaires' disease and more ordinary pneumonias are common after transplants (read chapter 8), as is tuberculosis (chapter 9). Aspergillosis is a common mold infection to watch out for. (Cancer patients are also at risk for this; see the preceding section on cancer.) Yeast infections from *Candida* and *Cryptococcus* and viral infections from herpes viruses are also common and are prevented in the same way they are in HIV-positive persons (see chapter 14).

You must avoid chickenpox the same way pregnant women do (see chapter 15), but do not get the new chickenpox vaccine—it is a live virus, and your immune system may not be able to contain it. A very rare bacterium called *Nocardia* sometimes invades after transplantation. It is found in decaying matter, so stay out of the garbage!

Toxoplasmosis, or "toxo," is a parasitic infection that you want to be sure not to pick up, if you don't already have it. Your blood can be tested for it. You get toxo from undercooked meat or from kitty litter (discussed more in chapters 14 and 15), but you can also get it from the organ given to you, especially if it's a heart. Toxo forms cysts in muscles and sits quietly there not bothering you. The heart is a muscle. If the transplanted heart has toxo cysts, they can start to grow again when you get started on your immune suppressing drugs. Usually your transplant team will look for it on your heart biopsies and start antibiotics if they find it.

Pneumocystis carinii is a parasite that causes pneumonia when given the opportunity of a weakened immune system. You cannot avoid exposure to it because it is already there in our lungs, usually quiescent. The best approach is to take medication to prevent it, preferably a sulfa drug like Septra. Your transplant team should include this in your medley of medicines. You can read more about it in chapter 14 because this is also the "AIDS pneumonia."

Perhaps the biggest infection problem in transplant patients is the cytomegalovirus, known as CMV. For mysterious reasons, this virus injures totally different parts of the body depending on the patient's condition. In AIDS (chapter 14), it targets the eye. In pregnancy (chapter 15) it targets the fetus. In heart transplant recipients it more often affects the stomach. In lung and bone marrow transplant recipients it tends to cause pneumonia.

If your blood tests positive for CMV before a transplant, the operation may reactivate your own quiescent virus, but this should not be a severe problem. If your blood tests show you are CMV-negative before a transplant, you must do what you can to stay that way. The most serious CMV infections are those in persons previously naive to the virus. First, you should only receive an organ or a blood transfusion that is also CMV-negative. Your transplant team will handle that. Next, you must not acquire a CMV infection from others. (You only get CMV from people.) Persons likely to transmit CMV to you are sexual partner(s) and children under two years of age. Pregnant women negative for CMV must also take precautions to avoid acquiring it (please see chapter 15).

With all these different things for a transplant recipient to worry about, it would be nice to know where to focus most of your attention at any given time. There is a very general pattern or time course to these infections laid out in figure 13.2.

No spleen

You will not be able to notice any difference if your gallbladder or your appendix is removed. It's almost the same for the spleen, until certain germs try to attack you.

Your spleen works like this: A large part of your blood, 4 percent per minute, is always circulating through your spleen. This blood slows down as it passes through a labyrinth of tunnels. There it is surrounded by immune cells that pick out bad apples. It's like quality control. It picks out bad red blood cells, foreign materials, and germs. The reason you can usually live quite well without your spleen is because there are other parts

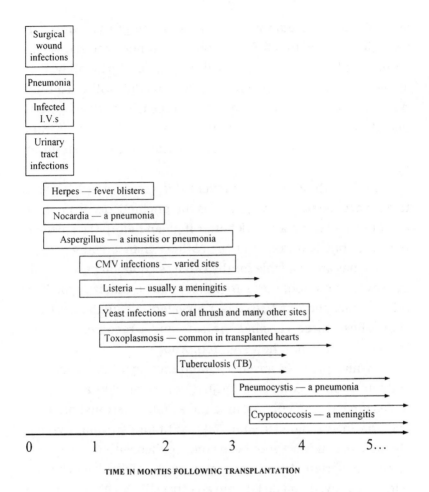

FIGURE 13.2 *The time course of infections following organ transplantation*

SOURCE: Adapted from R. H. Rubin, J. S. Wolfson, A. B. Cosimi, and N. E. Tolkoff-Rubin, "Infection in the Renal Transplant Recipient," *American Journal of Medicine* 70 (1981): 405.

of your body (the liver and bone marrow) that do the same thing. But when challenged by a hefty load of certain germs, the spleenless system gets overloaded and a serious infection results.

If you don't have a working spleen, the most important germ to watch out for is the pneumococcus, which can increase in your blood to incredibly large numbers and put you into irreversible shock within a few hours. Two other bacteria, *Hemophilus* and *Neisseria*, can be equally fatal, but, fortunately, they are less common than pneumococcus. An adult without a functioning spleen has only about a 2 percent chance of getting one of these infections. The risk is higher in children, or if the spleen was removed because of a disease rather than an injury.

The first thing to do to prevent this group of infections is to get vaccinated. The vaccine for the pneumococcus is called Pneumovax-23. It may work better if given before the spleen is removed, but just take it at the earliest chance you get to do so. Vaccines are available for the two less common bacteria that can invade you, too; these are *Hemophilus influenza* type B, or Hib vaccine, and, for *Neisseria*, polyvalent meningococcal vaccine. These three vaccines are safe and I recommend them highly. They are not, however, foolproof.

If your spleen is absent or nonfunctional, and you get a sudden fever, shaking chill, or just don't feel right all over, do not assume it is the flu. Assume the worst, that it just might be bacteria in the bloodstream. Take antibiotics promptly—you should ask your doctor to keep you supplied with the first dose of an appropriate drug. Then, call your doctor and get checked out right away. If you do fall into an especially high-risk category (for example, your spleen was removed because of Hodgkin's disease or has become nonfunctional because of sickle cell disease) your physician may want you to be on a preventive dose of penicillin every day. This is an individual decision.

Several even rarer germs can cause major havoc if the spleen is not there to protect you. One is a parasite called *Babesia*, which is transmitted the same way Lyme disease is. (Also read chapter 5 if you are at risk, and avoid high-risk areas for babesiosis if you can. These areas are Massachusetts's Nantucket

Island and Martha's Vineyard, and New York's Shelter Island and Fire Island.) Another worry for those without a spleen is a bacterium that is so rare that for a long time it did not even have a name. It is now called *Capnocytophaga canimorsus* and you get it after dog bites. Just be sure to see a knowledgeable physician promptly if you sustain a bite, and make sure everyone who treats you knows that you have no spleen.

Kidney failure

When your kidney function is poor enough to require dialysis (either washing the blood by using the kidney machine or by removing toxins through the abdomen with peritoneal dialysis), you become susceptible to infection in two ways. First, neither method of dialysis is perfect, and the toxins remaining in the blood can impede immune function. This makes you more susceptible to tuberculosis, which occurs ten times more frequently in persons with kidney failure than in everyone else. (Read chapter 9 well.) Another microbe, *Coccidioides* (or "cocci") is a fungus that is also more common in persons with kidney failure; it usually causes a TB-like pneumonia and is also a threat to HIV patients. It is discussed in chapters 8 and 14. With slowed urine flow, bacteria can build up in the urinary tract and cause UTIs. All you can do to prevent these is to drink plenty of water if you still make urine, always wipe from front to back after urinating if you are female, and get the urine checked out promptly if it turns cloudy in color or pungent in smell.

Second, the dialysis treatments can promote infection. If you are on hemodialysis (on a kidney machine) there is always a risk that bacteria on your skin could infect the fistula or graft the surgeon placed in your arm for blood vessel access. This is why dialysis nurses use strict sterile technique. Even so, the rate of infection in these fistulas and grafts runs to 2 percent or so per year. What you can do yourself is be sure there are no boils or other staph infections being spread around your household. (This is discussed in chapter 16.)

If the abdomen is being used for your dialysis (peritoneal dialysis), you will be doing most of the dialysis on your own. It has been shown that most abdominal infections (called peritonitis) on this type of dialysis are due to lapses in technique. When you are shown proper sterile technique by your nephrologist and/or dialysis nurse, it is important for you to follow every detail every time. When you err, bacteria or fungi will enter and grow in the abdominal cavity. This is a serious infection and can be very painful.

Liver disease

Chronic liver disease often scars the liver. Such scarring is called cirrhosis. One of the results of having cirrhosis is that the liver can no longer filter out bacteria that slip into your blood system from your bowels. This heightens your risk of food poisoning. In particular, you should avoid eating raw or undercooked shellfish altogether if you have liver disease. (See chapter 6 for more information on all kinds of food poisonings.) If two other complications of cirrhosis—bleeding from the stomach or intestines, and the buildup of abdominal fluid (ascites)—happen simultaneously, there is a high infection risk. The bleeding means that there is a break in the lining of the gut, and that break in the protective barrier allows bacteria to gain access to your system. When this double threat occurs you will want to be treated with antibiotics promptly.

Even without any gastrointestinal bleeding, ascites can become infected spontaneously. Bacteria can grow easily in abdominal fluid and cause an infection called peritonitis. Peritonitis is a serious and life-threatening complication of cirrhosis that may occur in up to one-quarter of persons with ascites due to chronic liver disease. At the University of Pittsburgh, Dr. Singh and his colleagues conducted a study with sixty people suffering from this condition. They gave thirty of these subjects trimethoprim-sulfamethoxazole (Septra or Bactrim), one double-strength tablet on Mondays and Fridays; the other thirty people (the control group) received a placebo pill. The results (published in 1995) were that only 3 percent of the treated persons developed an infection as compared with 30 percent of the control group. Septra is a sulfa drug that you might have an allergy to, but other antibiotics have worked prophylactically in this situation as well. Check with your doctor, but request this preventive approach.

Heart murmur

Our four heart valves direct blood through the heart in one-way flow and keep the blood from flowing backward. These tissue-thin, flexible structures let the blood flow through and then stop it so efficiently that someone listening with a stethoscope will ordinarily hear no sounds from the flow of blood. However, if a valve gets scarred, it can either become too tight or too stiff. If it gets too tight, only a narrow stream of blood can jet through the opening. If it gets too stiff, it won't close fully and a gush of backflow will occur with each heartbeat. In either case, the process is no longer silent, and a flowing sound called a murmur is audible. These abnormal streams also form eddies on the far side of the valves, and there the flow is sluggish. Tiny clots can form, and if bacteria enter the bloodstream they can become entrapped there and can set up an infection called endocarditis. It is a very serious infection because, as the heart pumps blood, the bacteria are launched into the bloodstream and spread everywhere else in the body. Moreover, the infection will further damage and can destroy the heart valve.

Persons who have had rheumatic fever in childhood often

have heart murmurs, as do many persons who were born with abnormal heart valves. The most common type of valve abnormality, mitral valve prolapse, also often causes a murmur. Although some murmurs that doctors designate "physiologic" or "innocent" are safe, other murmurs put you at risk for endocarditis. If you have a murmur (other than one deemed insignificant) and you are in a situation in which enough bacteria will be circulating in your blood to cause endocarditis, you will want to be on antibiotics.

When the dentist works on your teeth, the bacteria that normally reside in your mouth can enter the bloodstream and can cause endocarditis in people who are prone to it. In fact, mouth bacteria are the most common offenders. So, if you have a heart murmur, it is very important to take precautions. Make sure that the fact that you have a heart murmur is recorded on your dental records and remind the dentist at each visit. It hardly matters what the dentist will be doing; anything more than a simple examination qualifies; even a mere cleaning is risk enough. If you have a murmur and will be going to the dentist, get the correct antibiotics prescribed. (Antibiotic regimens recommended for the prevention of endocarditis are listed for you in appendix B. The pills can be prescribed by your dentist or your doctor; if you need an intravenous line [an I.V.], a doctor will generally handle this.) The first dose must be taken within one hour prior to the start of the dental work.

If your dental hygiene is poor or you have periodontal disease (bleeding of the gums), bacteria can sometimes get into your bloodstream without any dental procedure opening the way. If you are at risk for endocarditis, you must maintain the best oral hygiene possible, with regular brushing, flossing, and professional cleaning. You also should decrease the bacterial count in you mouth before all of these activities. The way you do this is by rinsing your mouth with a germicide called chlorhexidine (Peridex).

TABLE 13.3
When to take antibiotics to prevent endocarditis

Procedures presenting a significant risk to those with a heart murmur:

❑ Most dental procedures (any that could cause bleeding)

❑ Tonsillectomy or any other procedure in the respiratory tract

❑ Any procedure on the stomach or intestines

❑ Vaginal hysterectomies

❑ Any pelvic procedures in women if infection is present

❑ Any procedure on the urinary tract, even minor, including cystoscopy

❑ An operation for an infection, like draining an abscess

Exceptions, in which preventive antibiotics are probably unnecessary:

❑ A superficial dental exam

❑ An uncomplicated, normal delivery

❑ Placement or removal of an IUD

❑ Cardiac catheterization

❑ Endoscopy to look at the GI tract, as long as there's no surgery

❑ Bronchoscopy to look in the lungs, as long as there's no surgery

Many other medical or dental procedures can also force bacteria into your blood and may also require preventive antibiotics, but some other procedures are safe. See table 13.3.

Some people with heart murmurs have additional need to worry about endocarditis. If you have ever had endocarditis before or if you have a surgically implanted artificial valve, you have a major risk and want to be meticulous about prevention. The antibiotics of choice should be decided upon with your doctor. (Appendix B gives the American Heart Association's suggested list.)

Although we all face the risk of infection frequently in our lives, certain special situations magnify that risk. In this chapter I have addressed those unique hazards and explained how to negotiate them. Good luck!

14   *How to avoid infections if you have HIV*

*I*f you are HIV-positive, don't give in and don't give up. Even though, as yet, there is no cure for HIV infection or, when it later develops, AIDS, there is a lot you can do to extend life and to improve your quality of life. The most important thing to do is to understand what new infections you may have become susceptible to and learn how to avoid getting them in the first place.

Is it worth the effort? Yes. The cost of being apathetic here is high. First of all, the misery associated with some of these infections can be great. Take, for example one called "atypical TB," or *Mycobacterium avium* complex (MAC). We think you can now lessen your chances of getting this by 50 percent; that's lessening by half the chance of its associated night sweats, abdominal pain, and diarrhea. This in itself is worthwhile. You may also live longer. The secondary, or opportunistic, infections that HIV infection make you vulnerable to, can be fatal long before HIV alone would be. If you avoid getting the pneumonia of AIDS (*Pneumocystis*)—an achievable goal—you'll avoid your greatest risk of succumbing prematurely to a secondary infection. Another reason to work hard at prevention is that treatments for these infections are invariably worse than preventive tactics are. For example, a brain infection called toxoplasmosis can be prevented with a few pills taken two or three times weekly, whereas treatment involves an intrusive regimen of multiple medications. Lastly, picking up extra infections on top of HIV leads to a vicious cycle. When you get new infections, your immune system worsens significantly and you become even more susceptible to the next problem.

Let's go over some basic terms and concepts that will help you understand when you are at risk and what to do about that. Some of the microbes you need to concern yourself with are already present in your body, but are causing no harm. Efforts here are to prevent their "reactivation." You will want to find out through blood tests which of the pathogens you already have. Others pose a risk for you, but only because they are in the environment, and for these you want to learn to avoid "primary infection" or acquisition. No matter how these infections get started, if you are susceptible to them only because you have HIV, they are called "opportunistic infections" (OIs). That is, they can cause disease only when a faltering immune system opens a door for them. Preventing an OI before it ever happens is "primary prophylaxis," and preventing one from resurfacing is "secondary prophylaxis."

There are many ways to assess immune function. The most important one for persons with HIV is the CD4 count. This test counts an important immune cell in your blood that has several different names. It is called the CD4 cell, the helper cell, or T4 cell. (You may also hear the results of the test called the T-cell count or helper cell count.) The CD4 test is not perfect, and results can bounce around as much as 25 percent for no reason, but it is still the best gauge of immune status we have now. It will tell you when you become at risk for certain OIs and therefore when to take action. Because of its variability, often more than one reading is obtained before a major decision is made. But because of its central importance, the CD4 has become the basis for labeling the health status of people infected with HIV. The official dividing line between being just HIV-positive and having AIDS is a CD4 count of 200; those with fewer than 200 helper cells are said to have AIDS. (My sugges-

TABLE 14.1
How to use the CD4 count

CD4 result	When to get tested next	Why to get the test done
Over 500	6 months	Deciding whether to start anti-HIV treatments like AZT
250–500	4 months	Deciding when to start preventing *Pneumocystis*; assessing success of anti-HIV treatments
100–250	4 months	Deciding when to start preventing MAC infections; assessing success of anti-HIV treatments
Under 100	monthly	You should already be on an optimal anti-HIV regimen and a complete set of preventive strategies

tions for using the CD4 count to help you guide your care are given in table 14.1.)

HIV-specific therapy usually means taking two medicines in the nucleoside reverse transcriptase inhibitor (NRTI) class (e.g., AZT + 3TC) plus one more medicine in either the non-nucleoside reverse transcriptase inhibitor (NNRTI) class (e.g., efavirenz) or the protease inhibitor (PI) class (e.g., atazanavir). If you work with a knowledgeable HIV care provider and adhere to the regimen of three or more drugs that you mutually agree upon, your CD4 count will rise and your immune system can return to nearly normal. However, until then strategies to prevent specific opportunistic infections are at least as important, if not more important, than your anti-HIV therapy.

Literally hundreds of different kinds of viruses, bacteria, fungi, and parasites cause OIs. Fortunately, the list of common OIs is small, so preventive efforts can be targeted. The list of common OIs that are life threatening is even smaller: *Pneumocystis* (PCP), toxoplasmosis, *Mycobacterium avium* complex (MAC), and cytomegalovirus (CMV). Sometimes these are called "the big four."

For each of the sixteen most common infections that can cause an OI (including the big four), I will explain (in alphabetical order) what puts you at risk of catching it, how to avoid it in the first place, and, if you harbor it, what you can do to prevent it from making you ill.

Bacterial pneumonia

Ordinary bacterial pneumonia (as opposed to "AIDS pneumonia," or PCP, which is discussed below) is much more common in persons with HIV than in the general population. The risk of catching bacterial pneumonia becomes serious shortly after a person becomes HIV-positive, regardless of the CD4 cell count. (The whole of chapter 8, on how to prevent pneumonia, is worthwhile reading for anyone who is HIV-positive.)

The point to emphasize here is that there are three kinds of vaccines you should consider taking if you are HIV-infected: (1) pneumococcal (Pneumovax-23), (2) hemophilus type B or Hib (HibTITER), and (3) influenza vaccine. You only get the pneumococcal vaccine every six years; at worst, it may cause mild soreness in the arm and a low-grade fever. Hib is a similar vaccine for a less common pneumonia germ, but should be considered if you smoke or spend a lot of time around small children. Take the influenza vaccine yearly, around the first of November, not necessarily to avoid the flu, but to prevent the pneumonia that can follow it.

Candidiasis

Candida is a fungus—more specifically, a yeast—familiar to everyone. It is the same microorganism that causes diaper rash and the common vaginitis known as "yeast infection." It normally lives in our mouths, bowels, and genitals, but only causes a noticeable problem when its growth goes unchecked, as in AIDS. In AIDS it is pervasive; 90 percent of people with HIV go through at least one infection with *Candida*.

When candidiasis develops, the fungus produces a white coating on the membranes lining the tongue, throat, esophagus, or vagina. When it produces a white plaque on the tongue or throat, it is called thrush. When it causes vaginitis, a whitish discharge comes out of the vagina.

The fungus can also cause problems in parts of the body that are not visible to you. If it overgrows in the esophagus, the tube that connects the mouth to the stomach, swallowing food or drink will hurt, especially behind the breastbone. *Candida* esophagitis will also cause fever and weight loss. The good news, though, is that you'll often notice *Candida* first where it's easily identified, in the mouth or vagina, and you have an early opportunity to do something about it before it spreads.

Because *Candida* normally inhabits our bodies, you will never rid yourself of this fungus permanently. It is one of many infections that require careful control, rather than eradication. As soon as you first identify one episode of a yeast infection, maintain continuous control of it thereafter. There are two ways to do that. You can apply medicines right to the body surfaces involved (topical treatments), or you can take a pill that distributes the antifungal throughout the body. The local methods have fewer side effects, but are less convenient and will not prevent fungal infections other than *Candida*. I favor the pills for patients whose CD4 counts are less than 100 because they are at higher risk of other fungal infections, their yeast infection is more difficult to control, and because the side effects are really quite rare.

Topical treatment—either in the mouth or in the vagina—is best accomplished with clotrimazole (Mycelex, Lotromin) or nystatin (Mycostatin). These compounds are available without a prescription. After the yeast problem is controlled, monitor yourself closely for recurrence and start applying one of these medications again at the earliest sign of a relapse. If your doctor prescribes pills, the two commonly used are ketoconazole (Nizoral), 200 mg once daily on an empty stomach, and fluconazole (Diflucan), 100 mg once daily, at any time of day. Ketoconazole may inflame the liver (hepatitis) in very rare cases and may cause nausea. It may interact with other drugs, including some used for TB (INH and rifampin), seizures (phenytoin, Dilantin), and some drugs used for HIV itself. Diflucan can cause severe rash in rare cases and is more expensive. With either, you will run the risk of picking up fungi that are resistant to the drugs you are taking.

Cytomegalovirus (CMV)

Cytomegalovirus (CMV) is the most difficult of the big four OIs to control. Untreated, three-quarters of all people with HIV eventually get it. CMV was first cultured by virologists in 1956, and much work remains to be done before AIDS doctors and researchers (now sometimes called "HIVologists") will feel they have effective treatments for it.

CMV can cause infection in any organ system. And it causes unique syndromes in persons whose immune systems are handicapped in different ways. In people with HIV, it tends to strike the eyes, first causing blindness in one eye, and then—if not stopped—in the other. CMV affects other organs much less frequently. It can also injure the esophagus and the colon, causing pain on swallowing and abdominal pain. When CMV injures the nervous system, it may cause sudden difficulty walking and then paralysis.

When you first learn you have HIV, find out if CMV is already in your body. This is done by means of a blood test for CMV antibodies. If this test is positive, you have CMV but it may not presently be causing an infection. You are at risk for reactivation, however. If your test shows no CMV antibodies, you want to do all you can not to acquire CMV: if you are HIV-positive and pick up CMV for the first time, your chance of getting CVM disease is five times higher than that of an HIV-positive person who is at risk for reactivation.

If you are already infected with CMV, you need to watch closely for any evidence of disease. Your goal should be to get therapy very early. Have a baseline eye exam. This can be done by your HIVologist or by an ophthalmologist. Anytime you think there's any eye problem at all, go to the ophthalmologist. Their training in and knowledge of the retina is unmatched. If your CD4 count falls below 50, be particularly wary because this is when CMV retinitis generally occurs. As soon as CMV retinitis occurs and threatens your vision at all, medication should begin. Without adequate treatment, irreversible visual loss is inevitable. Unfortunately, both of the available therapies need to be started intravenously. Neither of them is curative and so treatment must be continued indefinitely.

In December 1994 the first pill effective against CMV, oral ganciclovir, was approved by the FDA, and it is being tested for prevention of retinitis. In one study, men with AIDS, a positive CMV blood test, and fewer than 100 CD4 cells were given either the drug or a placebo and then seen by the ophthalmologist monthly. The eye doctors found that 30 percent of those receiving the placebo had developed retinitis after eleven months, but only 16 percent of the treated group had. However, another similar study still in progress has shown no difference between the groups when it is left up to the patient to report a problem. I do not recommend preventive therapy with ganciclovir at this time because it offers no survival advantage, the drug is often toxic to the blood counts, you have to take more pills, and, if you fall into the group that fails therapy, you may be more likely to have a resistant viral strain.

If you are not yet infected with CMV, you want to do everything you can to prevent acquiring it. You acquire CMV from blood products and from body fluids of others who are shedding the virus. CMV can be found in any bodily secretions and is found in high levels in semen. If you test CMV-negative, therefore, it is imperative that you practice safe sex. (See chapter 10 for guidelines.) You have to assume that all adults are CMV-positive and remember that they may be secreting CMV-infected fluids at any time. In infants, CMV is commonly excreted in the urine for the first year of life. If you are at risk, ask others to handle diapers. If you need a blood transfusion and you are HIV-positive but CMV-negative, you should ask that the blood you are given be CMV-negative as well.

Coccidioidomycosis

Coccidioides immitis is a fungus, often just called "cocci," that is difficult for people with HIV to keep in check. It most commonly causes a pneumonia, but it can go anywhere in the body, often affecting the skin, joints, or bone, or causing a chronic form of meningitis. The good news about cocci is that it is geographically limited to areas of the West and the Southwest (see figure 8.1). Try to avoid going to those areas. If you must go there, be particularly careful when the desert dust blows. The fungal spores are often carried about on the wind, and you can catch coccidioidomycosis by inhaling the spores. If a dusty wind is brewing, you may want to wear a mask, or, better yet, go inside an air-conditioned building. If you live in high-risk areas—Tucson or Fresno, for example—take the same approach. You may also want to start taking an antifungal pill (see the section on *Candida*, above) once your CD4 count dips below 100, but the benefit of this is unproven.

Cryptococcosis

Cryptococcosis, a fungal infection, is on par with the big four life-threatening OIs for people with AIDS. (In the scientific literature *Cryptococcus neoformans* is the formal name of the fungus.) Both the disease and the fungus are called "crypto" for short. Crypto is one of the infections you acquire, rather than reactivate. Although little is known about how it is spread, it can be prevented with medications.

Crypto is drawn to the nervous symptom like a magnet. If you pick it up, you are most likely to experience fever, headache, neck stiffness, lethargy, and confusion. The bloodstream is its next most common site (fever, chills, malaise); lung infections (cough and shortness of breath) also occur. But cryptococcosis doesn't need to happen at all.

Cryptococcosis tends to occur when the CD4 count drops below 100. You don't get cryptococcosis from contact with other people, but you do probably breathe the fungus in. Most patients have no idea where they contracted it, but some seem to get it from close contact with birds. (Two crypto patients of mine raised birds.) Other than avoiding birds, people with AIDS have no way to be sure they are avoiding the fungus. So prophylactic antifungal medications can be used to prevent crypto. Dr. Edward Oldfield has shown that as little as one fluconazole (Diflucan) tablet per week is enough to ward off crypto, and Dr. David Rimland found that any patients of his who had been taking ketoconazole (Nizoral) didn't get crypto. The use of these medications is discussed under *Candida* above.

Diarrhea

Diarrhea is all too common in persons who are HIV-positive. It is a miserable bother but also more serious than many realize. In the United States, 30 to 59 percent of HIV-infected per-

TABLE 14.2
Opportunistic infections that cause diarrhea

Candidiasis (yeast)	HIV
Cryptosporidiosis	Isosporiasis
Cytomegalovirus (CMV)	Listeriosis
Giardiasis	Microsporidiosis
Herpes virus infection	*Mycobacterium avium* complex (MAC)
Histoplasmosis	Salmonellosis

sons will have a problem with gastroenteritis, while in the developing world 90 percent will. In Africa, AIDS is often called "slim disease" because of the characteristic severe weight loss brought about by chronic diarrhea; as the body loses fluids and fails to absorb nutrients properly, it wastes away. In people with HIV anywhere in the world, chronic diarrhea may be associated with severe dehydration, malnutrition, worsening of immune function, and heightened susceptibility to other OIs.

Diarrhea in AIDS is not always caused by infections. It can also be due to lactose (milk) intolerance, prescribed drugs, malfunction of the bowel's ability to absorb properly, or to HIV itself. But a long list of microbes may be responsible (see table 14.2). Fortunately, a single set of preventive measures can protect you against most of these diarrhea-causing infections.

The microbes that cause diarrhea enter your body through the mouth. If you are careful about what goes into your mouth—both on your hands and in your food and drink—you lessen your chances of picking up these infections. Some guidelines to follow: Cook all meats and poultry thoroughly. Avoid any farm-fresh foods; stick to store bought. Don't drink from lakes, streams, or other surface water. Never eat foods that have been allowed to sit out at room temperature for more than thirty minutes after their preparation. Take antacids and other acid-neutralizing medications only when needed (stomach acid provides a barrier to germs). Wash your hands often and thoroughly, especially before eating and after preparing raw foods, gardening, caring for small children, or handling animals.

Even if you follow all these suggestions faithfully, you cannot totally eliminate potential pathogens from what you eat and drink. Ordinary drinking water may sometimes contain some of them. In fact, in the United States in 1991 and 1992 seventeen states reported thirty-four outbreaks of illness due only to water intended for drinking; 17,464 persons were affected. If you act on the assumption that many kinds of food and drink might be contaminated—just as you should if you were traveling to the developing world, HIV-positive or -negative—then you might have a better chance of escaping the diarrhea of AIDS. Chapter 7 discusses in detail the question of what to eat and drink while traveling.

Two enteric illnesses deserve special mention because they are so serious. One is caused by *Salmonella* bacteria and the other by *Cryptosporidium*, a protozoan parasite.

Salmonellae are a group of bacteria that cause several different digestive tract illnesses, including typhoid fever. The most common kinds of *Salmonella* usually provoke diarrhea, fever, and abdominal cramps. Being HIV-positive makes you more than one hundred times more likely to get infected by *Salmonella*. The HIV infection also is apt to permit the *Salmonella* bacteria to move into the bloodstream, to cause prolonged illness, and to hasten relapse if antibiotic therapy is stopped. In order to avoid *Salmonella*, you should follow all the guidelines just mentioned and stay away from animals that carry it. Many animals may carry *Salmonella*, and there's no way to tell them apart from the safer ones that do not. Because *Salmonella* may survive for up to thirty months in animal feces, you have to assume that places where animals live may become contaminated. Reptiles can have carrier rates of 90 percent:

stay away from pet iguanas, lizards, and snakes. Turtles and ducklings also often carry it and cats may as well.

Cryptosporidiosis is also a major problem. We know relatively little about how to prevent it and less about how to treat it. It can cause diarrhea so severe and voluminous that it leads to shock. Patients with cryptosporidiosis experience profound weight loss.

You become infected by ingesting *Cryptosporidium* cysts. These microscopic cysts are highly infectious—as few as fifty of them can start an infection, and ingesting five hundred surely will. The cysts can be excreted from another person or be in drinking water or swimming pool water contaminated by the feces of small children. In one episode, eighteen AIDS patients contracted cryptosporidiosis on a hospital ward after one infected patient contaminated the ice machine. Although the federal Safe Drinking Water Act of 1974 specifies that cities must ensure the purity of their water, it does not require testing for *Cryptosporidium*. Outbreaks continue to occur in the United States, including one in Milwaukee in April 1993 in which 370,000 cases occurred and a number of AIDS patients died. Again, drinking only boiled, specially filtered, or bottled beverages may help prevent cryptosporidiosis (see chapter 7).

Hepatitis B

Avoiding hepatitis B is more important for persons with HIV than anyone else. If you are HIV-positive, you are nearly five times more likely than HIV-negative people to end up being a chronic carrier. Chapter 11 on hepatitis is essential reading for you. First, have your immunity checked. Because HIV and hepatitis B are transmitted in much the same ways, and hepatitis B is much easier to catch than HIV, many persons with HIV have already been infected with hepatitis B. But for those who show no evidence either of infection or immunity, getting vaccinated promptly is highly recommended.

Hepatitis C

We know less about the virus that causes hepatitis C, but it causes liver damage in even more cases than B. If you are HIV-positive, you should read the section of chapter 11 that deals with this disease, only receive blood transfusions when clearly necessary, and seek help if you inject drugs. If you are HIV-positive, have chronic hepatitis due to hepatitis C, but still have relatively intact immune function, you might be a candidate for antiviral treatment with alpha interferon. This series of injections might prevent hepatitis C virus from permanently damaging your liver.

Herpes simplex virus, Type 1 (oral) and Type 2 (genital)

It is difficult for HIV-infected persons to avoid herpes simplex virus (HSV) in the first place. Most people are infected with the oral form of HSV in childhood and most HIV-positive persons have already picked up the genital version before they get HIV. And there is no ridding yourself of viruses in this class—they stick with you for life. But HSV is actually one of the easiest of the opportunistic infections to control. A drug called acyclovir (Zovirax) puts HSV right back into a dormant and unrecognizable state.

Both types of HSV cause blisters and open sores. Type 1, the oral form, ordinarily causes lesions—"cold sores" or "fever blisters"—just outside the red of the lips, but in persons with immune dysfunction the sores can occur inside the mouth as well. Type 2, the genital form, usually develops on the penis in men and on the vulva in women. It also occurs quite often in the rectal area and between the buttocks. Most doctors, especially infectious disease physicians, can usually look quickly at these lesions and diagnose them on site.

The best approach to HSV is this: If you see any lesions at any time that are due to HSV, start acyclovir and don't stop. Acyclovir is known to be safe, even if taken for many years. A good dose to suppress HSV is 400 mg twice daily. Taken regularly, sores should be nonexistent or minimal. Good alternatives to acyclovir include famciclovir (Famvir) and valcacyclovir (Valtrex).

Herpes zoster

Herpes zoster is the medical term for the disease ordinarily called shingles. The shingles rash is caused by the same virus (varicella-zoster) that causes chickenpox. Years after someone has chickenpox, the virus—which has been harbored in the body all that time—somehow gets reactivated. It grows down a nerve root to the skin and causes a blistering rash to break out along the path of the nerve. So it, like HSV, causes blisters followed by sores. However, it occurs on one side only of the body or face.

Shingles can be one of the earliest manifestations of immune compromise from HIV. It does not signal advanced illness. Unfortunately, there is no known way to prevent shingles. But acyclovir—given as 800 mg five times a day—can shorten the course of zoster when it happens. Start within seventy-two hours of onset. Famvir and Valtrex work, too.

Histoplasmosis

Histoplasmosis is another serious fungal infection. It is caused by *Histoplasma capsulatum*, nicknamed "histo." Like cocci, it is found in soil and has a limited range. This one's a

Midwesterner. It occurs in a band centered around the Ohio and Mississippi valleys, extending approximately one state over in either direction from the rivers. It is also found in some areas of the Caribbean and South America. Histo is often seen in Indianapolis, Kansas City, Memphis, Puerto Rico, and the Dominican Republic, or in persons who've moved from these areas. Whereas histo develops in only one of two hundred persons with AIDS nationwide, one in four of those in the Midwest and Caribbean gets it. These are the people who must consider special precautions.

Histoplasmosis in persons with AIDS may be totally different than the chronic TB-like pneumonia seen in persons whose immune systems are intact. If your CD4 count is below 100 you are at risk for "disseminated histoplasmosis," which, as the name suggests, affects many different parts of the body. It most commonly starts over days to weeks and causes high fever, weight loss, cough, shortness of breath, and enlargement of the liver, spleen, and lymph nodes.

You get histo by inhaling the spores of the fungus, which enjoys an unusual niche in our world: guano. The droppings of birds harbor it, and those of bats, also. If you are HIV-positive you will want to stay clear of bird roost sites, caves frequented by bats, barns, and construction and remodeling sites where spores of histo are likely to be suspended in the air.

There is no proven primary prophylactic medication for histo. Two experimental trials failed to show any benefit in taking antifungus pills. But if you live in a histo zone and have a CD4 count under 100, you might consider asking your doctor to check your blood for histo on a regular basis and start therapy as soon as it shows up on a test. One medication called itraconazole (Sporanox) is more potent against histo than the others, but whether it will make a good prevention drug is not yet known.

Mycobacterium avium **complex**

Mycobacterium avium complex is a particular form of atypical TB, not to be confused with TB itself. It is called MAC (formerly MAI) for short. Although it rarely affects people whose immune systems are healthy, it has a strikingly high incidence in people whose CD4 cells are under 100; their chances of acquiring a MAC infection in a given year are one in five.

Although MAC can be treated (with a multidrug regimen), it can also be pure misery. It is a common cause of drenching night sweats, fever, fatigue, weight loss, diarrhea, abdominal pain, malabsorption of food, and profound anemia.

MAC is common because the bacterium is ubiquitous in the environment: it can grow in ordinary tap water, and it is a normal resident of soil. Although there is no way to avoid the bacterium of MAC, you can do something to lower the chance of getting the infection. Under the direction of Dr. Beverly Wynne of the Adria Corporation, many doctors (including myself) gave patients with AIDS—close to five hundred people, altogether— either an antibiotic active against MAC or a placebo, not knowing if preventive treatment would work or side effects would be troubling. As it turned out, MAC developed half as frequently in the treatment group and side effects were minimal. These days, however, even better MAC-prevention drugs have been found. If your CD4 count is under 100, take either azithromycin (Zithromax) 1,200 mg (two pills) once a week or clarithromycin (Biaxin) 500 mg (one pill) once a day.

Pneumocystis carinii **pneumonia**

Pneumocystis carinii pneumonia, usually called "PCP," is the worst of the big four infections of AIDS. This is because of its frequency and its severity. As many as three-quarters of persons with AIDS get PCP; it is often the first indication that they are infected with HIV.

Pneumocystis pneumonia starts slowly and develops over weeks or months. Its symptoms include fever, cough, chest pain, and shortness of breath, first on exertion and later at rest. PCP is caused by a one-celled parasite, *Pneumocystis carinii*, which lives, in low numbers, in the lungs of most people. Given the opportunity—in this case a CD4 count under 250—it begins to multiply and cause pneumonia. *Pneumocystis* will only rarely infect any other part of the body.

Thank goodness there is effective prophylaxis for PCP and that it is generally easy to take. If you are HIV-positive and have a CD4 count of less than 250, start PCP prophylaxis promptly, and don't stop. From my own medical practice, I can tell you that many cases occur when the preventive treatment is not followed faithfully. Off treatment, 40 percent of HIV-positive persons at risk will get PCP per year.

The most effective thing to take is also the easiest. Trimethoprim in combination with sulfamethoxazole, sold as Septra or Bactrim, is the treatment of choice. To prevent PCP (and toxoplasmosis), take one double-strength tablet once a day three days a week or one regular tablet daily. It's not expensive. The antibiotic will markedly diminish your risk of contracting PCP almost to zero.

The problem with this sulfa drug is that many persons become allergic to it. Most allergies show up in the first three months. About one-third of the HIV-positive people who take it have side effects: nausea and vomiting, rash, fever, and diarrhea. If you are one of those who cannot tolerate Septra, work closely with your HIVologist to choose the best alternative for you. These include dapsone, 100 mg by mouth daily, and liquid atovaquone (Mepron) 750 mg in 10 ml, or two teaspoons, daily. A breathing treatment with 300 mg of pentamidine (Pentam) monthly was popular but has fallen out of favor because it does not work as well as the other options and may promote certain respiratory infections. However, presently, nothing seems to compare with the trimethroprim-sulfamethoxazole combination. Therefore, with increasing success (over 50 percent), many allergic patients are being desensitized to the drug. They take very small doses at first and build it up slowly according to a defined schedule that any HIVologist will have a version of for you.

Syphilis

If you are practicing safe sex (discussed in detail in chapter 10) you should not acquire a new case of syphilis. However, syphilis can be a silent disease for years, and you need to know if you've ever picked it up in the past. Fortunately, there's an easy blood test for it. As soon as it is determined you are HIV-infected, your doctor will want to run this test on you and thoroughly treat any syphilis found before it surfaces and causes illness. Get retested yearly. If, at any point, your syphilis test is positive, you may need to have a spinal tap (lumbar puncture) done, because if it shows that the syphilis spirochete has entered the nervous system, you will need a more intensive approach to treatment and monitoring.

Toxoplasmosis

The fourth major life-threatening infection of AIDS, toxoplasmosis, is called "toxo" for short. It affects 5 to 10 percent of AIDS patients and is the most common brain infection they suffer. It usually starts with fever and headache and may lead to seizures and weakness as well. The microbe that causes this one is a one-celled organism, a protozoan.

Toxoplasmosis infections are common but the disease is rare. Most people do not even know they have been infected. However, if your CD4 count falls below 200 and you are harboring toxo, your chances are almost one in three of getting the disease. And this is the way it usually happens: toxo is already present in your body and then it reactivates. Although they are much less common, primary toxo infections do occur and tend to cause more severe problems than the reactivated illness does. It is best to make sure neither reactivation nor initial infection happens, and you can do this.

First, determine if you are already infected by having a simple blood test for antibodies to *Toxoplasma*. If they are present, the toxo protozoan is in your body somewhere, although you wouldn't know it otherwise. If there are no toxo antibodies in your serum, you've never picked it up, and you are much less likely to ever have a problem with it.

If you are lucky and are free of toxo, you will want to take several precautions in order to stay that way. Adults get toxo by eating the protozoan's cysts. There are two sources of cysts: they can be excreted by cats or found in meat. Cats are the natural host of toxoplasmosis and do not become noticeably ill from it. However, at any given time one in a hundred cats is excreting toxo cysts in its feces. Since you cannot pick these cats out, assume any cat may be a source. Give the job of changing a cat's litter box to someone who is HIV-negative. If you must do the job yourself, do it daily because the cysts take some time to become infectious outside the cat's body; wear disposable gloves and wash carefully afterward. Sterilize the pan occasionally with bleach or disinfectant. Cats may leave their feces in the garden and in children's sandboxes as well. Wear gloves when working in such places and wash up right afterward.

Toxo cysts are common in the meats we eat. To avoid ingesting the live cysts, cook the meat thoroughly—to at least 66°C (150°F), to be exact. Smoking and curing kills the cysts, too, and frozen meats are generally safe. Wash your hands after cooking. Don't have drinks made with raw eggs, another occasional source of cysts (as well as *Salmonella*).

If you already have toxoplasmosis in its silent, inactive form, there is no way to rid yourself of it. About 25 percent of American adults fall into this category. (It is more common in Europeans; 90 percent of French people have it by age thirty.) But you still don't have to get sick with toxoplasmosis. The way to prevent it is with medication. When you become at risk—when your helper cells are below 100—start the treatment. Conveniently, the same regimen that is best for *Pneumocystis* (PCP), another protozoan, works to avert toxo. Three to seven double-strength trimethoprim-sulfamethoxazole (Septra DS) tablets taken over the course of each week are effective. If you are allergic to sulfa, as many people are, an alternate regimen is one 50-mg or 100-mg dapsone tablet daily and one 50-mg dose of pyrimethamine (Daraprim) once weekly. This prevents PCP as well.

Tuberculosis

If you become HIV-positive, your chances of getting tuberculosis go up markedly. You are also more likely to have a case that spreads throughout your body. And you are more likely to infect people around you. Chapter 9 gives plenty of advice about how not to get TB in the first place. Please read it, and ask the people who live with you to read it, too. The methods outlined in that chapter are not always foolproof, though. Fortunately, it is also possible for you to take preventive medications, and they generally work, even when your immune system is compromised. However, these medications can have side effects, so you only want to take them if you need them.

Consider yourself at heightened risk for TB if your CD4 count has fallen to 500 or less. At that point, start prophylactic INH if there's any indication at all that you may have picked up the TB bacillus (see table 14.3). The details on INH and TB skin testing are given in chapter 9. You should have a skin test at least yearly. A panel of extra skin tests—ones that you are expected to respond to—should be included to make sure that

TABLE 14.3
Precautions against TB for people with HIV

*Persons with HIV should take preventive medicine for TB
(if they haven't been previously treated) if:*

1. The PPD skin test gives a 5-mm reaction, now or ever before.

2. They cannot respond to any skin tests and live in a country or community where TB is very prevalent.

3. They use drugs intravenously (and thus have a much higher risk of TB).

4. They have been exposed to anyone with tuberculosis (regular TB, not atypical TB or MAC).

you are indeed able to respond to a skin test. If you don't respond to one of those, the PPD could be falsely negative. Get your first test as soon as you find out you are HIV-positive. The higher your CD4 count, the more likely your body will react appropriately to the skin testing material. Ninety-eight percent of people whose CD4 count is over 800 will respond to the test, while only 40 percent of people whose count is under 200 respond. If the test is positive, you have a one in three chance of getting TB within two years, but you can nearly eliminate that risk by taking the INH.

Recently, TB bacteria resistant to INH and other drugs have emerged. And the majority of persons with these strains of TB have been HIV-positive. These multidrug-resistant strains make tuberculosis all the more frightening. They are not only more difficult to treat than ordinary TB, but are highly contagious. So far, this kind of TB is centered in the New York City and Miami areas. It is there that you need to be most careful about avoiding potential exposures. Let's say you find out you've been exposed to a strain of TB resistant to INH. The CDC (and I) recommend a preventive drug regimen for you involving two or three other TB medicines. You can get these from your regular doctor or from the Public Health Department (at no charge). I should note that the effectiveness of such a regimen has not yet been demonstrated conclusively. (See table 14.4 for a summary of the foregoing.)

Other things you can do

There are a number of other things you can do that, although not specific for any particular infection, may give you a better chance of avoiding OIs (see table 14.5). Eat well! In particular, eat a high-protein diet. Protein and calories are needed to produce immune cells; undernutrition is definitely associated with decline in immune function. (That's one reason why famine and infectious disease are so closely linked.) If you have a well-balanced diet of at least 1,200 calories per day, you will be eating plenty of vitamins in your food, but an additional multivitamin per day won't hurt. Exercise, particularly aerobic exercise, has been shown to raise CD4 counts, in addition to its other physical and psychological benefits.

Some kinds of behaviors—smoking, injecting drugs, and unprotected sexual activity—encourage opportunistic infections. Smoking is known to be associated with a more rapid decline in CD4 counts. It leads to respiratory infections in persons with normal immune systems, and is even more likely to do so in persons with HIV. Injecting drugs lowers the immune system's ability to ward off infections and permits infections to get worse quickly. Drugs also impair the user's ability to follow preventive strategies and prescribed treatments, and they increase the chances that HIV and other infections will spread to others. Unprotected sex, even between two HIV-positive persons, can not only transfer the germs that cause OIs but can also transmit HIV strains. One partner might contract a new strain that is more virulent and/or more drug-resistant than the one he or she already has.

Persons infected with HIV can also help themselves by always learning, always asking questions, and by actively participating in their own care.

TABLE 14.4
Things to take to prevent opportunistic infections

Candidiasis:

You are at risk if you see any thrush or have any vaginitis.

Best medicine: topical clotrimazole (Mycelex) troches or nystatin (Mycostatin) if CD4 > 100 and ketoconazole (Nizoral) or fluconazole (Diflucan) pills if CD4 < 100.

Cryptococcosis:

You are at risk if your CD4 count is < 100.

Best medicine: fluconazole (Diflucan) 100 mg once daily or ketoconazole (Nizoral) 200 mg once daily.

Cytomegalovirus infection:

You are at risk if your CD4 count is < 100.

Best medicine: none yet.

Hemophilus infection:

You are at risk if you are HIV-positive, especially if you smoke.

Best medicine: Hib vaccine once; yearly influenza vaccine.

Hepatitis B:

You are at risk if your blood tests show no past or present infection.

Best medicine: Hepatitis B vaccine.

Hepatitis C:

You are at risk if blood test show you are not already infected.

Best medicine: none.

Herpes virus infection:

You are at risk if you've ever in the past had herpes.

Best medicine: acyclovir (Zovirax) 400 mg twice daily.

Histoplasmosis:

You are at risk if you live in the Midwest and your CD4 is less than 100.

Best medicine: none yet.

Mycobacterium avium complex (MAC):

You are at risk if your CD4 is less than 100.

Best medicine: azithromycin 1,200 mg once weekly.

Pneumococcal pneumonia:

You are at risk if you are HIV-positive.

Best medicine: pneumococcal vaccine (Pneumovax-23) at diagnosis and influenza vaccine yearly.

TABLE 14.4 (*continued*)
Things to take to prevent opportunistic infections

Toxoplasmosis:

You are at risk if your blood test is positive for toxo and your CD4 is less than 100.

Best medicine: trimethoprim-sulfamethoxazole (Septra, Bactrim), three double-strength tablets per week.

Alternate: dapsone 100 mg daily and pyrimethamine (Daraprim) 50 mg weekly with folinic acid (Leucovorin) 25 mg weekly.

Tuberculosis:

You are at risk if you have a positive (more than 5-mm) PPD skin test, exposure to a known case, or do not react to skin tests and live in a community with a very high rate of TB.

Best medicine: isoniazid (INH) 300 mg daily with pyridoxine (vitamin B_6) 25–50 mg daily, for at least one year.

TABLE 14.5
Things to do to prevent opportunistic infections

1. Maintain a high-protein diet.
2. Eat only fully cooked meat and poultry.
3. Drink only bottled or previously boiled beverages, and consume no drinks containing raw eggs or unpasteurized milk.
4. After cooking, wash your hands thoroughly.
5. Avoid kitty litter and places where cats mess.
6. Avoid caves, bird roosts, and demolition sites.
7. Practice safe sex.
8. Get aerobic exercise at least thrice weekly.
9. Avoid persons with colds, flus, and chronic coughs.
10. Review your itinerary with a specialist at least a month before travel.
11. Always continue to ask, learn, and be willing to modify your approach.

15   *If you are pregnant*

When I was a boy, my father's friends were fond of telling me, "I knew you when you were just a twinkle in your father's eye." This quip implied not only the father's passion for the mother but also for the unborn child. It also implied that a pregnancy was planned, or at least might have been anticipated. This is when caring and protecting children should begin—well before they even are conceived.

At conception, when the sperm and egg join, the entire new being is only one cell. If any injury occurs to that cell, the entire organism is damaged. It begins to grow and in only about thirty hours it pinches off to become two cells. Damage now would hurt at least half the developing fetus. In another three days it has become sixteen cells, and so on. In these early stages, before the mother can even be aware she is pregnant, injury is generally fatal and a miscarriage occurs. But you can see that, in general, the earlier in pregnancy a fetus gets hurt, the more it may be damaged. Therefore, the time to start planning to protect your child is when you just have that twinkle in your eye.

The developing fetus can be injured in several ways. An accident can cause physical trauma. A nutritional deficiency can hinder development. (Eat plenty of fresh greens when contemplating pregnancy to keep your folic acid levels up. This vitamin is needed for the spinal column to form properly.) But the most insidious threat to the unborn is infection.

Many infections can cause malformations in your unborn child. It is natural to fear these infections not only because they can cause severe disabilities but also because these particular infections are all around you. Two potential avenues of infection are especially worth noting. First, expectant mothers often spend time around children, and several of these infections are primarily transmitted by children. Second, to become pregnant, by definition you have to be sexually active, and another group of germs that can pass to the fetus are sexually transmitted. Read this chapter carefully, either before getting pregnant or as early in gestation as possible, to find out how you can minimize the risk of serious infection in your unborn child.

Protecting the child is only half the reason to avoid infections during pregnancy. The mother is at risk as well. When you are pregnant, you have a compromised immune system. To some extent, the fetus is foreign material to you and the immune system's job is to expel foreign material. So, the immune system is turned down a notch during gestation. Also, the hormonal and physical changes that accompany pregnancy slow the normal flushing action of fluids through your body. All these changes put mother at risk for some serious infections we will discuss.

Physicians often refer to the most important infections affecting pregnant women by the acronym TORCH. These letters stand for toxoplasmosis, other, rubella (German measles), cytomegalovirus, and herpes. In the "other" category, syphilis, HIV-1 (the AIDS virus), listeriosis, group B streptococcus, hepatitis B, and urinary tract infections are all important. Each of these can be prevented. I will tell you how. We'll start with the "T-RCH" infections and then move on to the "O" category. Table 15.1 summarizes the basic information.

Toxoplasmosis

This parasite is a real menace, but utterly avoidable. About three thousand infants are born infected with toxoplasmosis

---

TABLE 15.1
Basic rules for the expectant mother

---

1. Start following these rules as soon as you consider becoming pregnant.

2. Adjust your diet:
   a. Eat only well-done meat, poultry, and fish.
   b. Wash all vegetables thoroughly.
   c. Consume no soft cheeses, deli counter foods, unpasteurized milk, or raw eggs.
   d. Wash your hands after cooking.

3. Do not change kitty litter yourself.

4. Wear gloves when you work in the garden; then wash your hands.

5. Avoid anyone with a fever, new rash, new arthritis, or swollen glands.

6. Remain monogamous during pregnancy; if your sexual partner has CMV or herpes he should wear condoms.

7. If you are not immune to rubella, get vaccinated during a menstrual period and practice birth control for three months thereafter.

8. If your blood test is negative for CMV (you are susceptible): avoid intimate contact with children under two and keep susceptible children away from day care as much as possible.

9. If you have ever had genital herpes, tell your obstetrician and come to the hospital early, as soon as labor starts.

10. Get tested, and treated if necessary, for syphilis, chlamydia, gonorrhea, urinary tract infection, and vaginitis.

11. Get tested for hepatitis B and alert your pediatrician if the test is positive.

12. Have cultures for group B streptococcus done in your last 3–6 weeks to see if I.V. antibiotics will be needed at delivery.

---

in the United States each year, and many more in other countries. The risk that a mother with this infection will pass it on to her child varies with the stage of her pregnancy. If toxoplasmosis is acquired before conception, it is rare for the fetus to get it, and even if acquired before the tenth week of pregnancy, it is unlikely for the infection to cross the placenta. However, the further along in pregnancy you are, the more likely it is that the baby will also become infected: 30 percent for the second trimester, and 60 percent for the third. Conversely, the earlier the parasite does make it across to the fetus, the more damaged the fetus will become.

Mothers who become infected with toxoplasmosis usually feel well, or merely have a flulike illness, but they may have fever, swollen glands, rash, and enlargement of the liver and spleen. Affected children can suffer a range of symptoms, usually involving the nervous system, varying from low IQ scores, to visual or hearing defects, to severe brain defects.

You can transmit toxoplasmosis ("toxo," for short) to your fetus only if you pick it up for the first time during your pregnancy. If you've previously contracted it, as have about one-fourth of adults in the United States, you don't have to worry. You can find out your susceptibility by having a simple blood test done. If you are susceptible, or don't know, use the following guidelines to avoid getting it.

Humans get infected by ingesting toxo cysts. The cysts are found in two places. First, any materials contaminated with cats' excrement can be infectious. The cat is the natural host of this microbe and cats are excreting cysts 1 percent of the time. The second place you find toxo cysts is in undercooked meats. So, here's what to do. If you have a cat, don't allow it outside where it might pick up toxoplasmosis. Do not clean a cat's litter box yourself. Someone else will need to do it—and do it daily, so as not to give the cysts a chance to mature. Wear gloves when you work in other places where cats leave feces, such as sandboxes and gardens; when you are through, put the gloves in the laundry and wash your hands. Control flies and cockroaches.

Cook all meat thoroughly; this will inactivate any cysts, which cannot be seen with the naked eye. When cooking, do not taste raw food; clean counters and utensils promptly, and wash your hands before and after cooking. Eggs can also transmit toxo. Consume no food or drink that could have been made with raw eggs. Eating frequently outside the home is another risk factor for toxoplasmosis, probably because you have less knowledge of and control over what you eat.

If for any reason you think you might have contracted toxo, the situation is not by any means hopeless. Tell your doctors right away; they can verify your infection and then start giving you a special antibiotic, spiramycin. Spiramycin is safe in pregnancy but may be cumbersome to obtain because it requires a special request to the Food and Drug Administration.

If blood tests do show you have contracted toxoplasmosis during pregnancy, an amniocentesis and extraction of fetal blood can be done to determine whether the infection has passed the placenta to the fetus. If it has, your doctor may want to use more potent drugs, sulfadiazine (Microsulfon) and pyrimethamine (Daraprim). The French have a national program to control congenital toxoplasmosis. They have shown that treatment is effective: the newborns who received treatment as fetuses are usually normal.

Rubella

German measles is a cruel infection for the unborn. Of the fetuses who are exposed to the rubella virus, 10 to 20 percent of them will be severely damaged or malformed. The worst problems occur early in pregnancy; after twenty weeks there is little risk of malformation. Before twenty weeks, the congenital anomalies that can occur are wide-ranging. If the rubella virus infects the fetus before twelve weeks, heart deformities are most common; at twelve to sixteen weeks, deafness is often associated; later in pregnancy, dysfunction of the eye, ear, and/or nervous system is common, but the problems are usually less severe.

Fortunately, congenital rubella syndrome is now very rare and easily prevented. Total elimination of congenital rubella might really happen one day. After an epidemic in 1964, thousands of infants were born with the congenital rubella syndrome; the first vaccine was licensed in 1969. Now this country is down to only twenty cases per year. You should ensure that you are immune to rubella before you conceive. Rubella vaccine is your key tool for avoiding this problem. Before you get pregnant be sure you have been properly vaccinated.

If you received a rubella vaccine anytime in your life after your first birthday, consider yourself immune. Hopefully, you have records of your immunizations. The rubella shot has been part of the standard childhood vaccination series since 1970. If you served in the military, you were vaccinated. If there is any question, get a blood test done. If it shows that there are any antibodies to rubella, you know you are immune.

If you are not immune to rubella, get vaccinated. The vaccine is a live virus vaccine and so is theoretically harmful to the unborn child. To be on the safe side, take the vaccine during a menstrual period. After that, do not get pregnant for three months. The vaccine is safe, but in adult females who are not yet immune, it can have side effects. You may get joint pains and mild arthritis—temporarily—after vaccination.

If you find yourself pregnant and not immune, you will want to avoid anyone with a fever plus rash, arthritis, and/or swollen glands. Rubella is hard for doctors to diagnose, but those are the symptoms an infectious person would have. Rubella is contagious starting five days before the rash begins and until seven days after that. After delivery, get vaccinated promptly.

Cytomegalovirus

Cytomegalovirus infection (CMV) is the most common congenital infection: 1 percent of all children in this country are infected with CMV, or about forty thousand newborns per year. Fortunately, the infection is usually unnoticeable, even to their parents. Nine out of ten of the infected infants are normal at birth, but 10 percent, or four thousand in the United States yearly, have some problems. This smaller group may be seriously infected with major abnormalities of the brain, eyes, ears, liver, and blood. Another 10 percent of them are normal at birth, but have relatively minor problems later. My son is one of these. He is now an honor student and a talented soccer player, but when he was an infant he had an inguinal hernia and what we called his "brown tooth," one without enamel. These are two of the most typical abnormalities of mild CMV. Some problems with vision and hearing may also occur later in childhood.

I cannot give you advice that will eliminate CMV from your life—half of us are infected with it already. CMV is one of those viruses that are ubiquitous, and, once incorporated into your cells, it stays with you. However, you can indeed learn to prevent the serious manifestations of CMV. These only occur in newborns of mothers who become newly infected just before or during pregnancy. So start by having a blood test for CMV antibodies to see if you are already infected. If you are among the 50 percent of adults who have already contracted CMV, you can breathe a little sigh of relief. Your unborn is not at risk for serious forms of CMV disease, and there is really nothing for you to do. But, if you do not have these antibodies circulating in your blood, you will want to pay close attention to ways you can avoid acquiring CMV during pregnancy. As it stands now, two in a hundred women do get CMV during those forty weeks.

You get CMV from another person who is shedding the virus. Usually it is transmitted through oral secretion (from saliva, a cough, a sneeze), but urine (changing diapers) and genital secretions (sex) can spread the virus as well. If your blood test shows you are susceptible, you will want to avoid intimate contact with those around you who may be shedding it, specifically, certain infants and men.

Small children commonly excrete CMV for the first two years of life. For example, Dr. Stuart Adler of Richmond, Virginia, checked the kids attending day care in his city, and a full quarter of them were shedding the virus in their urine or saliva. If you have a previous child who is still under two, you may want to have that child tested for CMV as well. This can be done on a finger prick sample of blood. If that child's blood test is positive, you must assume he or she may be contagious: avoid mouth-to-mouth contact, wear gloves when handling diapers or respiratory secretions, and wash your hands frequently. (Unless the older sibling has spent time in day care, this situation, where the child is already infected but the mother is not, will be unusual.)

For older CMV-negative siblings, try to avoid day care and other close contact with other small children. For both you and this child, contact with kids over two is okay. If your job involves children, try to be assigned to older ones. If you are a nurse, following the usual "universal precautions" for hospital personnel will be very important, especially on pediatric, cancer, and AIDS wards.

Get your husband or any regular sexual partner tested also. If that person is either positive or untested, and you are negative, use condoms during sex and avoid mouth-to-mouth contact. Remain monogamous during pregnancy.

Herpes

Genital herpes virus (HSV) infection is very common, but it is quite rare these days for a fetus or newborn to contract it. Of those who do become infected, though, 70 percent will die. You have to be very careful about genital herpes. The most common way the baby is infected is when a previously infected mother is shedding virus from her cervix at the time the baby passes through it during labor. But a much more dangerous situation, and one that is more easily preventable, is when the mother has a primary (first-time) infection. I'll discuss that first.

If you've never had a genital herpes virus infection, you certainly do not want to start one up while you are pregnant or intending to become pregnant. It is only these primary infections, not the more common recurrent infections, that can cross the placenta and infect the fetus. The infection is usually fatal. Fetuses that survive may have severe eye and brain damage and skin scars. How to avoid picking up primary HSV is discussed in chapter 10 and if you've never had genital herpes, read it well. Suffice it to say here that if you have never had it, but your sexual partner has, he should wear a condom during sex for the duration of your pregnancy. See chapter 10 for directions for the proper use of the male latex condom.

If you've already had a case of genital herpes, ever, you may reactivate the infection at any time. You are right to be concerned about transferring the virus to your baby. Fortunately, you and your doctor can make sure your baby is born uninfected. You must tell your obstetrician that you have had genital herpes and make sure that information is repeated as you get close to delivery. There is no way of predicting whether you will be producing HSV at the time you ultimately deliver. Neither a previous positive culture nor a previous outbreak during pregnancy makes it any more likely that you'll be contagious at the time of delivery. No matter what happens during the nine months of pregnancy, your chance of reactivating on the day of your baby's birth runs about 1.6 percent. So, plan to enter the delivery suite early to allow time for a detailed examination.

If by experience you have learned that certain sensations, such as an itchy, prickly feeling in the genital area, signal an outbreak and it's happening then, be sure to tell your doctor. (The medical term for such an early warning sign is prodrome.) If you feel there's an eruption brewing or your doctor actually finds one, a cesarean section should be done. This should be done *before* your membranes rupture (that is, before the water breaks).

Even if all goes well and there is no indication of a problem, request that "screening cultures" be done. This set of cultures will tell if there were viruses being produced at delivery, even though they had not formed a visible lesion. If positive, the pediatrician and/or neonatologist will look the baby over carefully and possibly start the appropriate antiviral drug.

No amount of care on your part or that of an obstetrician can totally eliminate the chance of passing HSV to the infant. Since the known cases are now handled with extreme care, most of the infections now happen when the mother had no prior knowledge she had herpes. Modern medicine has not yet learned how to detect these cases. You should still feel quite safe, though. The rate of neonatal herpes runs only about 4 in 100,000 births. It is now a rare infection.

"Others"

Syphilis. Syphilis is different from most congenital infections. The later in pregnancy it occurs, the higher the chance that it will cross the placenta and injure the fetus. This gives you extra time to make sure you are not carrying syphilis. Part of every first prenatal visit is a blood test for syphilis, usually an RPR. If this is positive, you should be treated with an antibiotic that can both kill the syphilis bacteria, *Treponema pallidum,* and also cross through the placenta and into the fetus where it is needed. Intravenous or intramuscular penicillin is the preferred treatment.

After treatment, get monthly blood tests throughout the rest of your pregnancy and review them with your doctor to make sure the therapy worked. If you (or your sexual partner) do not remain monogamous during pregnancy and have any unprotected sex, you must inform your obstetrician and get tested again late in pregnancy and at delivery. If you do this, you can still receive antibiotics and avert congenital syphilis in the child, which can cause deafness, hydrocephalus, and mental retardation, among other problems.

Hepatitis B. The hepatitis B virus is easily transferred by intimate, direct contact. The birth process is just that. If you are infectious for hepatitis B, there is a 90 percent chance your baby will catch it during delivery. And getting this virus at birth is worse than getting it later in life. (See chapter 11 for a detailed explanation of hepatitis B.) One in four of the children who do contract it at birth will ultimately, decades later, develop a scarred, functionless liver (cirrhosis) or, worse yet, liver cancer. Fortunately, there are tools available to stop this dreaded virus before it has a chance to do any damage to the young one.

To find out if you carry the hepatitis B virus, you should take the hepatitis B surface antigen (HbsAg) blood test. Have it performed anytime during your pregnancy. This test by itself is enough, but your doctor may also want to run a test called HbeAg to find out if you're highly infectious or not. If your HBsAg is positive, your baby should be treated shortly after delivery.

Within twelve hours of birth the newborn receives both a shot of supercharged globulin (designated HBIG) and a first shot of vaccine. Be sure the vaccine series is completed on schedule at one, two, and twelve months of age. This therapy is quite safe. In fact, it has been made part of the ordinary childhood routine. (But if the mother is infected, it starts early.) If your baby receives each of these therapies, the chance of the baby developing hepatitis B is reduced by 90 to 95 percent.

Group B streptococcus. Streptococci are bacteria that make their home in and on us and generally do not bother us. There are hundreds of kinds and they each favor different parts of us as their home. Group B streptococci (*Streptococcus aga-*

lactiae) reside in the vagina and rectum. This means that your baby is not unlikely to acquire these germs as it is born. Many do. Unfortunately, their immune systems cannot control this germ and each year up to ten thousand babies in the United States get seriously infected with group B streptococci. About two thousand of these children die. About 10 percent of the infected children get meningitis and, if they survive this complication, are likely to end up with severe brain damage, delayed development, and/or learning disabilities. Fortunately, this infection is preventable. And here's how.

Not all mothers carry group B streptococci, and it can come and go. The best test for it is a culture. Samples are collected from both the cervix and the rectum with cotton swabs. If you have these cultures taken within six weeks of delivery, they will predict fairly well whether you'll be carrying group B streptococci at the time you give birth. If you are, you can take antibiotics and prevent your child from contracting the infection. In doing this, you'll be helping yourself as well. Mothers get infected with group B strep, too. It may contaminate your uterus or a surgical wound, and it is a not uncommon cause of fever after childbirth.

Some programs offer preventive antibiotics only to the mother-infant pairs at highest risk—premature deliveries (over three weeks early), premature rupture of membranes (broken waters more than twelve hours before delivery), and mothers with fever. However, 80 percent of the time with group B strep infection high-risk factors are lacking and the pregnancy is otherwise normal. So, if either of your screening cultures are positive, you will want to insist on prevention, even if all's going well in your pregnancy. Cultures are repeated near delivery, but you'll most likely start on intravenous antibiotics while you are awaiting the results. Ampicillin, a kind of penicillin that works effectively against group B streptococci, is normally used, but erythromycin or clindamycin (Cleocin) can be given if you're allergic to penicillin. They are started at least an hour before delivery to allow enough time for the medicine to reach all of your blood, the amniotic fluid surrounding the fetus, and the blood going through the umbilical cord to the fetus. If cultures at delivery come back negative, therapy is stopped; if they are positive, a course of antibiotics is completed. These extra efforts pay off!

Listeriosis. Listeriosis infection is rare in humans. Veterinarians who care for farm animals, however, are very familiar with it. They know it as "circling disease" because of the way it affects a cow's nervous system. The infection also commonly causes miscarriages in cows, sheep, and goats. When listeriosis occurs in people, it is often epidemic. The epidemics occur because many people eat the same contaminated food. And the contamination is usually from an animal source. In Halifax, Nova Scotia, in 1981, contaminated coleslaw caused a large outbreak. The cabbage came from a farm on which two sheep had died of listeriosis, and the farmer used sheep manure to fertilize his cabbage fields. In Boston in 1979 an outbreak was traced to a garnish of raw vegetables that presumably had been fertilized with contaminated compost. In 1983 in Massachusetts a specific brand of milk was the culprit. The dairy cows had listeriosis.

Listeria monocytogenes, the microbe that causes listeriosis, grows just fine in the refrigerator, and pasteurization may be inadequate to kill it. One very large epidemic—in Los Angeles in 1985—implicated a specific brand of Mexican soft cheese. Contamination of the cheese with unpasteurized milk probably led to the outbreak. In Switzerland in 1987 it was soft cheese again; in Philadelphia in 1987 it was ice cream and salami; California broiler chickens in 1992; and pork in France in 1993. On the very day I was writing this chapter a recall of honey-cured ham was announced on the radio. The report said it was because of contamination by a little-known bacterium called *Listeria monocytogenes*. Outbreaks continue.

In these epidemics, pregnant women, fetuses, and infants are affected far out of proportion to their numbers in the population. They will account for more than half of the infections. The risk is greater in the last third of pregnancy. Typically, weeks (not just days) after ingestion, fever and a flulike illness with headache and muscle aches begin. The infection usually does not become severe or life-threatening to the mother. But within three to seven days the uterus and fetus may become infected, which leads to premature labor and loss of the baby. Since listeriosis has a long incubation period, infection may not be apparent at birth; the infection may not show up in the newborn for days or weeks. It is a serious and life-threatening infection in these very young children.

Listeriosis does not always occur in epidemics, however. In fact, sporadic cases outnumber those in the outbreaks. They are food-related as well, and generally are associated with soft cheeses, undercooked poultry and hot dogs, and food purchased from delicatessens.

There are three things you can do to prevent the ravages of listeriosis: (1) be aware of epidemics; (2) be careful what you eat; and (3) get treated promptly if you think you may have contracted it.

Call your local health department and ask if there is an outbreak going on. Thoroughly cook all meats (especially hot dogs), and wash all vegetables completely. Do not eat soft cheeses like Mexican-style, blue, Camembert, Roquefort, and Brie, but cream cheese and hard cheeses are okay. You may want to avoid deli food during your pregnancy as well. If you get a new fever during late pregnancy and have any reason to suspect *Listeria*, contact your obstetrician (and possibly an infectious disease specialist) promptly. Antibiotics can be given to prevent the spread to your baby. Only about one baby in ten thousand in the United States will get listeriosis, but don't let it be one of yours.

Other "Others." There is a smattering of other mother-child infections that are either quite rare or less serious than the usual TORCH infections. They are, however, worthy of keeping an eye out for, so I'll mention each briefly.

Fifth disease is a childhood illness caused by parvovirus B19. It got its odd name from its place on an antiquated list of childhood infections with rash. (The disease was first recognized in the nineteenth century.) Children with this minor infection get a fever followed by a typical rash. The parvovirus rash has a "slapped cheek" appearance. Children with such red faces are no longer contagious. Stay clear of any setting in which fifth disease is being seen, though. Parvovirus B19 can cause miscarriage and a serious anemia in newborns. Older children can develop a serious anemia as well, and they remain infectious.

Chlamydia trachomatis is the most common of the sexually transmitted diseases (see chapter 10). If mother is a carrier, neonates can contract it as they are born and get lung and eye infections. Just to be sure, get tested, and treated if necessary. You can safely do both anytime during your pregnancy.

Measles (red measles or rubeola) in a pregnant woman can cause malformations in the fetus and premature birth. Although measles vaccinations have been standard practice since 1963, measles outbreaks still occasionally occur, especially on college campuses. The best policy is to be sure of your immune status before conceiving. If you know you've had measles or have had two vaccinations after 1967, you are immune. Otherwise, update your measles vaccine three months or more *before* conceiving. (Do not get the vaccine if you are already pregnant.) If you find yourself susceptible to measles and exposed during pregnancy, you should receive a gamma globulin injection within seventy-two hours. This may prevent or at least ameliorate the problem.

Lyme disease may be able to harm a fetus, and I go over this in detail in chapter 5.

Some kinds of *malaria* can infect a fetus and cause premature delivery or miscarriage. Unfortunately, the best medicines for preventing malaria are not safe during pregnancy. You will do best to stay out of malarial zones for the nine months. See chapter 7 for more details.

AIDS (HIV) is an infection every woman needs to be aware of before and during pregnancy. In the United States, women accounted for 9 percent of the first hundred thousand cases and 12 percent of the next hundred thousand. In my practice in 2003, women accounted for 22 percent of the HIV-positive cases. In Africa, where the epidemic has matured, half of the victims are women. Of women infected with HIV in the United States, 80 percent are in their reproductive years, and six thousand HIV-positive women give birth in this country every year. Read chapter 12 on HIV and AIDS carefully.

Illnesses that are harder on moms

Until now I have been urging you to be wary about infections primarily on your child's behalf. Now I need to tell you about two infections that can be as risky for the mother as for her child. They are chickenpox and urinary tract infections.

Chickenpox. Over 80 percent of U.S. citizens have had chickenpox (varicella) by age ten, and you usually only get it once. Of the people who don't remember having it, 80 percent really did and are immune. However, some people do slip through to adulthood without being exposed, and about one in every two thousand pregnant women gets chickenpox. When this happens, the baby runs only a 2 percent chance of being injured by the virus in the first half of pregnancy, and an even lower risk later. Rarely, if infected in the first half of pregnancy, a child can be born with a shrunken arm or leg, or exhibit a range of nervous system abnormalities; if infected late in pregnancy, only a scar on an extremity may occur. However, the expectant mother runs a substantial risk of severe disease and life-threatening chickenpox pneumonia.

Chickenpox can occur year round, but is particularly prevalent in late winter and early spring. At any time, if you think you have never had chickenpox, do not be in the same room with anyone who might be contagious. This virus travels through the air. A person is contagious for chickenpox from up to a few days before the rash starts until about a week after that. You come down with it just about two weeks after you've been exposed. If you do find yourself exposed, get blood tests promptly to see if you're really susceptible or not. If you are, get treated with a special globulin available to prevent it: varicella zoster immune globulin (VZIg). This injection is effective if it is given within ninety-six hours of exposure. In the worst case—you're pregnant and you get chickenpox—your doctors may want to treat you with an antibiotic active against varicella: acyclovir (Zovirax). Doctors do not like to give it during pregnancy, but so far it has not been shown to be harmful to the unborn.

If you plan far enough in advance, you can avoid the chickenpox issue altogether by getting vaccinated. If you have never had chickenpox—or if you're not certain—request that your blood be tested for varicella antibodies. If you already have antibodies, you are immune. If you do not have antibodies, avail yourself of the new chickenpox vaccine (discussed in chapter 4 and appendix A), but do not become pregnant for three months after the shot. It is a live-virus vaccine and its effects on a fetus are entirely unknown.

Urinary Tract Infection. Many women get frequent urinary tract infections (UTI), usually just in the bladder. The female anatomy favors this kind of problem, and if you are expecting, you are even more prone than usual. This is because the normal flow of urine, which provides a flushing action for the urinary tract, is slowed. Hormones make the urine-carrying tubes lax and the growing fetus pushes on them. Although UTIs can be associated with small newborns and premature births, the mother is at greater risk of getting a bad and sometimes life-threatening infection up in the kidney (pyelonephritis).

The best approach is to have your urine cultured when you first find out you are pregnant, even if you have no urinary symptoms. This has become part of routine prenatal care. If

TABLE 15.2
Getting tested during pregnancy

	Test	Source	Timing
Tests all pregnant women should have	CMV serology	Blood	First visit
	Syphilis serology (RPR)	Blood	First visit
	Urine culture	Urine	First visit
	Group B streptococcus cultures	Cervix, rectum	Last 3–6 weeks
	HIV serology	Blood	Before 12 weeks
	Chlamydia antigen	Cervix	Anytime
	Gonococcal antigen	Cervix	Anytime
	Hepatitis B surface antigen (HBsAg)	Blood	Anytime
Tests some pregnant women might need or want	Herpes culture	Lesion	Diagnosis unknown
	Listeria cultures	Blood	If suspected
	Rubella serology	Blood	Anytime
	Toxoplasmosis serology	Blood	Anytime
	Varicella antibody	Blood	If exposed

the urine has significant numbers of bacteria, you stand a one in four chance of getting a kidney infection during pregnancy. If you get treated with appropriate antibiotic pills (preferably for two weeks), you will avoid pyelonephritis. Reinfections occur up to 35 percent of the time, so get cultured again at each of your monthly checkups thereafter.

Although the microbial world poses many dangers for mother and fetus, a systematic approach to prenatal care will prevent problems. Table 15.1 summarizes the infection-preventing techniques for you. Table 15.2 gives you a list of the tests you should insist on having. When your healthy child is delivered, you will consider all this time and effort a worthy investment.

16 *In the hospital*

We enter a hospital to mend one ill, and ironically we may contract another. Often the new malady is an infection. This problem of hospital-acquired infection is huge (see table 16.1). Its costs can be counted in dollars and extra hospital days, but the distress of patients who get setbacks instead of cures is immeasurable.

There are many reasons you might become infected in the hospital. The most important reason is that your body's natural barriers to infectious microorganisms get violated. For example, your largest and most important barrier to infection is your skin; but if you have surgery or just need an I.V., the wound in your skin is an open door to germs. Your urethra normally keeps bacteria out of your bladder and kidneys, but when hospitalization requires a tube (a Foley catheter) to drain urine, bacteria can find an easy way in.

Stomach acid kills many germs before they reach your gastrointestinal tract, but antacid medications are commonly given in hospitals. A natural gateway near the vocal cords closes off the lungs to germs, but if you require a ventilator this door is kept open. When something does go down your windpipe, you cough it out, but in the hospital pain medicines, sleeping pills, or your own weakness can make it difficult to cough effectively.

In the hospital, moreover, just when your illness makes you extra vulnerable, you are exposed to the most virulent and hard-to-treat germs we know. Hospital germs are heavyweights. And some of them are nearly unique to the hospital environment. These include the most resistant types of *Staphylococcus, Streptococcus,* and TB. Each year bacteria grow more resistant to

TABLE 16.1
The costs and risks of hospital-acquired infections

Infection type	Extra hospital days	Extra charges (1992 dollars)	Chance of dying	
			Direct	Contributing factor
Bloodstream	7.4	$3,517	4.4%	8.6%
Pneumonia	5.9	$5,683	3.1%	10.1%
Urinary	1.0	$ 680	0.1%	0.7%
Wound infection	7.3	$3,152	0.6%	1.9%
Others	4.8	$1,617	0.8%	2.5%
Total (average)	**4.0**	**$2,100**	**0.9%**	**2.5%**

SOURCE: Centers for Disease Control, "Public Focus: Surveillance, Prevention and Control of Nosocomial Infections," *Morbidity and Mortality Weekly Reports* 41 (1992): 783.

antibiotics. Recently, several strains of bacteria have emerged in hospitals that are resistant to nearly all known antibiotics. A *Streptococcus* called vancomycin-resistant *Enterococcus* is one of these and multidrug-resistant *Pseudomonas aerugenosa* is another. When these germs invade, they can be fatal because no good treatment is at hand.

If you need major surgery or your vital signs are unstable, you may need the acute care and keen observation available only in hospitals. But, if your tests and treatments can be done safely out of the hospital, you're much better off. Besides avoiding contact with all those hospital germs, being treated as an outpatient is less costly. Besides, most patients tell me they get more rest at home.

More and more services are being made available for outpatients. In the past, some medical tests required you to stay in the hospital for a couple of days. That is very rarely the case now. Physical therapy, intravenous fluids, medications, chemotherapy, nursing, x-ray, and many surgical procedures are now available in the home or clinic setting. Take advantage of them.

If you must enter the hospital, you will be at risk primarily for four types of infection: wound, lung (pneumonia), urinary tract, and bloodstream. You *can* help out as a patient (or family member) to prevent these. I'll go through each type of infection one by one and give you some tips on prevention.

Wounds

An open wound is an open invitation for bacteria. Keep them out! First, don't take the *Staphylococcus* bacteria to the hospital with you, especially if you will have surgery. It loves to grow in wounds. You will know if you are carrying staph if you have one of the skin infections it causes. They are commonly called boils, but any skin or nose infection that holds white or yellow pus, from a drop to a cupful, is probably a staph infection. Once staph is on you, it often stays for years. It also spreads to other family members who may or may not get boils. A recent patient of mine had a terrible time with a staphylococcal abscess on her lower back after the neurosurgeon removed a slipped disk. She had not had boils before this, but her son had. When I cultured her nose (which appeared normal), there were the staph bacteria. In one study, the presence of staph in the patient's nose before cardiac bypass surgery increased the risk of getting a wound infection by ten times.

If surgery is planned for you or a family member, and if any one of you has had boils or another staphylococcal infection anytime in the last three years, get your nose cultured for staph. If it is positive, a cream called mupirocin (Bactroban), applied liberally four times a day for a week, will clear it. Also, bathing or showering with a germicidal soap, like Hibiclens, for about a week before the procedure, will get the staph off your skin. Pay extra attention to body creases. The effort pays off.

Once in the hospital, you want to keep those treacherous new germs off your body. (This is a worthy goal whether you will have an open wound or not.) When germs first take up residence on us (the lingo is "colonize" us), there are no signs that they are present. They bide their time until an opening for infection occurs. If you don't let them gain this initial foothold, they won't infect you.

Most of the time, hospital germs are deposited on you by the hands of hospital care workers. If one of these well-meaning people touches another patient or contaminated materials and picks up the harmful bacteria on his or her hand, the bacteria will stay there for over two hours. A doctor, nurse, or technician can touch many individuals during those two hours and pass on the bacteria to any or all of them.

All this has been known for a long time. In the nineteenth century a Hungarian physician, Ignaz Phillipp Semmelweis, found that too many women on his maternity ward in Vienna were dying of "childbed fever." He theorized that the doctors were passing it from mother to mother, and ordered them to wash their hands thoroughly between patients in a solution of chlorinated lime. The epidemic, which we now know was caused by a strep bacterium, halted. (Semmelweis himself later died of a strep infection.) This sort of thing still happens today.

In a perfect world, all hospital personnel would wash their hands before and after every patient contact and wear gloves whenever touching a wound. They are trained in this way. Nevertheless, in actual practice, hospital care workers wash hands or don fresh gloves less than half as often as they should, even when coaxed and cajoled to do so.

If hospital committees don't ensure compliance with hygiene measures, you be the guard. If you go about it the right way, you'll gain more respect than scorn from those caring for you. Try polite but straightforward reminders, such as "I've read I can get an infection just from being touched. Would you mind washing your hands before you help me?" and "If you're looking for the gloves, they're in the dispenser on the wall."

Also, beware of the hospital worker who enters the room already wearing gloves. It's easy for a doctor or a nurse in a hurry to forget to change gloves between patients. It's also easy for hospital workers to absentmindedly rub their nose or scratch a skin eruption after washing their hands. If they are carrying staph, the previous hand washing won't help you avoid the germs. Be the watchdog for your loved ones if they are too ill, too young, or too old to do so for themselves.

Pneumonia

Pneumonia has been dubbed "the messenger of the angel of death" because it is a not uncommon terminal event for a person who is already seriously ill. I've devoted a whole chapter (chapter 8) of this book to pneumonia. But, if you find yourself in the hospital and it's not yet time for your angel, fight back. The main way to prevent hospital-acquired pneumonia is not to allow respiratory tract secretions to stagnate. A constant flushing of the airways is essential. In fact, doctors inelegantly dub this "maintaining pulmonary toilet." So even if it hurts, even if you've had chest surgery, even if you're sleepy from pain medications, keep coughing.

There are many reasons why your cough reflexes can be dulled when you are ill and medicated, so you may actually need to keep a schedule. If necessary, make an appointment with yourself to go through a series of deep breathing and coughing every fifteen or thirty minutes. If needed, respiratory therapists may be called in to help you. They have special ways to promote effective coughing. Getting up and out of bed as much as possible helps, too.

Another favor you can do yourself when you enter the hospital, especially if you are going to have surgery, is to stop smoking. Smoking stimulates the production of mucus, and you'll have to cough all the more to get it out. Stop smoking as far beforehand as you can, so the extra mucus production slows down. Smoking also hinders blood circulation. So, by stopping smoking, you give your heart and blood vessels the chance to work at their best. It can make a big difference to the rate of healing.

Urinary tract infection

UTIs are common infections in the hospital. The Foley catheter—a tube inserted into the bladder that allows the free flow of urine into a bag—is a very helpful device. It's essential when you are too weak or lethargic to go to the bathroom, after you've had pelvic surgery, or when your physician needs a precise measurement of your output. But it also is like an escalator for bacteria. It permits them to move easily up to the bladder and kidneys.

When the catheter is no longer needed, you want it out. Requesting the removal of a Foley catheter is the single most important thing you can do to prevent hospital-acquired UTIs. If you're male and you still can't get out of bed, you may be ready to use a hand-held jug; request a "urinal." If you're female, you might consider the bedpan demeaning and inconvenient, but UTIs are certain if the Foley stays in long enough, and they can be serious. Even diapers or intermittently inserting catheters to drain the bladder are preferable to leaving one in continually.

If you must leave the Foley catheter in, watch the urine in the tubing that runs between the catheter and the collection bag. Urine is normally transparent. If it develops a sediment, that may be a sign of infection. The urine should be checked in the lab, and any infection should be treated before you develop a high fever or worse.

Bloodstream infections

Most bloodstream infections in the hospital (actually 86 percent of them) are related to intravenous lines. Think of it: an I.V. provides a pathway from your surrounding environment, to your skin, to your blood, and from there to every inch of your body. And the bacteria take advantage of it, too. It's a scary thought. There is a significant chance of dying from these infections (see table 16.1). In addition to contamination at the catheter insertion site, occasionally problems occur when contaminated solutions are run through the I.V. or a nonsterile line is inserted (see figure 16.1).

In view of all these risks, extra care is given to sterile technique in dealing with intravenous lines and medications. Most

Although a catheter can be contaminated from a number of sources, the patient's own skin appears to be the largest source of infection-causing microorganisms.

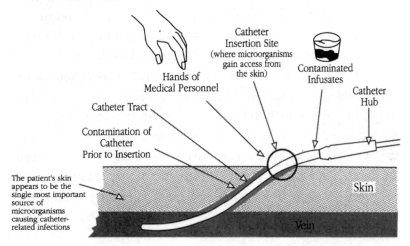

FIGURE 16.1 *Sources of infection from intravenous lines*
Bacteria are given multiple opportunities to gain access to your bloodstream when you have an I.V. Although a catheter can be contaminated from a number of sources, the patient's own skin appears to be the largest cource of germs.
Source: Arrow International, Inc.

TABLE 16.2
Diseases that can be transmitted by blood transfusion

Babesiosis	*Malaria*
CMV	Parvovirus B19
Hepatitis A	? Prion diseases
Hepatitis B	*Trepanosoma cruzii* (Chagas disease)
Hepatitis C	Trypanosomiasis
HIV	West Nile virus
HTLV I and II	Yersinia

hospitals have specific teams designated to deal just with your I.V.s, and they follow strict guidelines and routines for insertion and maintenance of the catheters. All medications intended to go through them are mixed in absolutely antiseptic environments. Despite all this, I.V.-related bloodstream infections occur frequently, accounting for 16 percent of all hospital-acquired infections.

What can you do for yourself or your family member to decrease the risk of bloodstream infection? Again, be on patrol. Watch for and report redness, pain, swelling, or drainage at the site where the needle enters the skin. If you have no fever, these changes might just be from the irritation of the chemicals going into the vein, from a reaction to the catheter itself, or from a catheter that is missing the vein. But if you have a fever, they may indicate an infection that is only going to get worse. In either case, report those changes to your regular nurse, your I.V. nurse, or your doctor. If you are getting I.V.s at home, the same holds true—and make sure the dressing over the entry site remains intact. Never touch that area with your hands.

Blood transfusions

Getting a blood transfusion in the United States is safer than ever. Before transfusion, blood is tested for no less than seven infections, including syphilis, hepatitis B, hepatitis C, HIV-1, HIV-2 (a rarer cause of AIDS), HTLV-1, and HTLV-2 (HIV-like viruses). But testing is not foolproof and some risk remains whenever you need to take in blood products. I have listed all the infections one may be at risk of from a blood transfusion in table 16.2.

Since AIDS is the biggest worry after blood transfusions, please look at chapter 12, where I discuss how to avoid getting a blood transfusion in the first place.

The hospital is truly a place where lives are saved. It is also, despite the best efforts of hospital workers, an unsterile environment and a danger zone for infection. I hope that you never need this advice. But if you do, I hope that it helps you get the best care the hospital can offer and brings you out again unscathed by infection.

Five

Twenty-first-century infections

17   *Emerging infections*

*T*he microbial world is constantly springing surprises. Germs evolve, adapt, and migrate, finding new ways to prosper in their hosts. When humans are their host, we become alarmed, and appropriately so. Infections that are new to us are more virulent; they are attacking an immune system that is unprepared.

These new host-parasite struggles are termed "emerging infections." An emerging infectious disease is one that is new to us in some way. SARS, for example, is entirely new, caused by a previously unknown virus. Contrast this with West Nile virus, which is an emerging pathogen only because it moved. Long known to the Old World, it seems that West Nile virus took an airplane to La Guardia airport in the summer of 1999. Mad cow disease and avian influenza ("bird flu") emerged by jumping to a new species—humans. Many different bacteria have become emerging pathogens, reinventing themselves by mutating, thereby becoming resistant to antibiotics or producing a new toxin. Germs employ many different techniques to evolve and advance themselves, constantly surprising us with new threats and forcing us to be more creative in devising new ways to protect ourselves.

West Nile virus

The story of the discovery of West Nile virus in the New World is a story of astuteness, serendipity, and perspicacity. In August 1999, Dr. D. Asnis of Flushing Hospital, Queens, N.Y. was astute when he found it unusual that he had two patients at the same time with viral encephalitis. He contacted the New York City Department of Health and quickly six additional cases were identified, all in northern Queens. It was serendipitous that a Chilean flamingo died that month in the Bronx Zoo. This alerted veterinarians in New York, and it turned out that many nearby crows were dying as well. One perspicacious veterinarian, Dr. Tracey McNamara, pointed out to her human-treating counterparts that the viruses that cause encephalitis in the United States do not normally kill birds. Epidemiologists, like all good scientists, try to follow the principle of Occam's razor ("among competing hypotheses, favor the simplest one"), so they reasoned that perhaps both the human and the bird epidemics could be blamed on the same agent. If this were the case, they needed to look for viruses that originated elsewhere. By September 1999, West Nile virus had been identified in both species. This was the first time that this virus had been found in the Americas.

West Nile virus is new to us in the United States, but it is not a new virus. It was first discovered in the blood of a woman with fever in the West Nile district of Uganda in 1937. For many years, West Nile virus has prospered in the Eastern Hemisphere where it routinely causes outbreaks. One measure of its long history in Europe, Asia, and Africa is that West Nile fever rarely kills birds in the Old World. Given time, the virus has developed a nonlethal relationship with its usual vertebrate host, the bird. This relationship is better for both parasite and host alike. But since its introduction to North America, where this relationship has not had time to develop, crows have been dying in droves.

What about people? More and more of us are being exposed to the West Nile virus as time goes on. In the first year the virus visited us, sixty-two persons in New York City were hospitalized because of West Nile fever and seven of them died from

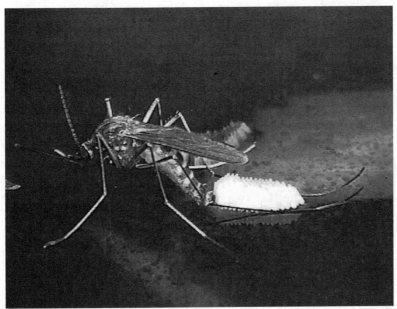

FIGURE 17.1
A *Culex pipiens* mosquito laying her eggs. Eggs such as these may already
be infected with West Nile virus.
Source: Centers for Disease Control and Prevention.

it. The virus spread quickly and blood tests taken by the CDC
indicated that over two thousand people contracted the virus
in the year 2000. Then the virus began to spread down the East
Coast and reached Florida. Later, it traveled westward. By 2004,
there had been over nine thousand confirmed cases and over
two hundred deaths: it had spread across the entire country.
Colorado, Nebraska, and the Dakotas had the most cases, probably because the dryer climate of the upper Midwest is most
favorable for *Culex* mosquitoes, the genus that transmits the
virus most efficiently. The single most common species that
acts as a vector for West Nile virus is *Culex pipiens*, commonly
called the Northern House Mosquito (see figure 17.1).

Why so many infections and so few deaths? Only certain
individuals are very susceptible to the deadly forms of West

Nile virus infection. The following case history offers a painful illustration.

One Saturday morning in August 2002, I was called to the emergency department to see an eighty-two-year-old woman with a fever. Her temperature was 103.8 degrees. Since she was abnormally groggy, I had to get the story from her daughter.

The patient lived alone in a residential area of the city of Atlanta and loved to garden. She told her daughter five days earlier that she had found a dead blue jay in the yard and discarded it. For the last two days she had a flulike illness. Her daughter went to check on her this particular Saturday morning and found her quite ill.

The woman looked very ill to me, as well. She was very weak, difficult to arouse, and her neck was somewhat stiff. We wanted to rule out meningitis right away, but we needed to do a brain scan first to make sure it was safe to do a spinal tap. The brain scan was normal. The spinal tap was not; it suggested a mild viral infection of the central nervous system. Her disease was not mild, though—she was dead by Sunday night.

By Sunday it had become obvious that although the spinal fluid was mildly affected, the brain was where the bulk of the problem lay. The patient was loosing all brain function, including her drive to breathe. Her daughter pointed out that she had a living will and did not want to be placed on a ventilator. The West Nile antibody tests run on blood and spinal fluid were not reported to us for two weeks because the laboratories at that time were so backed up with requests from all over the country. But when we finally received the results, they were all strongly positive. When West Nile fever leads to encephalitis it is a devastating disease.

It is the older individual who is most at risk from serious illness and death from West Nile virus. In the 2002 epidemic in the United States, the average age of all confirmed cases was fifty-five years. The average age of those who died was seventy-eight years. You can develop West Nile fever at any age, but you are much more likely to become seriously ill if you are over fifty years old. Overall, 1 in 150 infections results in the most serious manifestations: meningitis and encephalitis. Compared with children, the risk of these life-threatening nervous system complications is ten times higher if you are in your fifties and over forty times higher if you are eighty years of age or older.

The older we get, the more important it is for us to take precautions. These precautions include avoiding mosquito bites from May until the first frost, but especially in August and September, when West Nile fever is most common. In chapter 7, I have listed the basic techniques for avoiding mosquito bites. Here are some more specifics: When you are outdoors, wear pale colors. Bright colors, as well as cologne or jewelry, may attract insects. Clothing should cover and be loose since insects can bite right through tight garments. While clothes should be long and loose, they should be of thin material because staying cool diminishes the risk of attracting biting insects.

Eliminate mosquito breeding grounds from your environment. Mosquitoes lay their eggs in stagnant water. Historically, the puddle of water inside discarded tires has been a favorite breeding site for mosquitoes near human habitation. In 1900, Dr. Walter Reed and others proved, partly through self-experimentation, that yellow fever was transmitted by the bite of a mosquito. Shortly thereafter, Dr. William C. Gorgas was able to rid Havana of the disease by eliminating mosquito-breeding habitats. When work on the Panama Canal slowed to a crawl in 1904 because workers were constantly ill from yellow fever and malaria, Gorgas set out again to control these diseases by clearing brush where mosquitoes swarmed and draining swamps where they bred. Gorgas's greatest impact may have been the result of removing countless old tires from the Canal Zone.

In our place and times, we have a different set of mosquito

havens. Store empty flowerpots upside down. When in use, be sure they drain well. Lay out-of-door wheelbarrows and garden tools in any way that will allow water to drain from them after rain. Consider draining birdbaths and deny mosquitoes small puddles of water wherever you may find them. If there is a collection of water that you choose not to eliminate, such as a decorative fountain or fishpond, you might consider treating it in the spring with a larvicide.

Larvicides either kill mosquitoes shortly after they hatch or they prevent their maturation into adults. (It is the adult mosquito that bites and transmits West Nile virus.) Methoprene is one available larvicide. It is nontoxic to birds and mammals, but may kill shrimp and crabs and is moderately toxic to fish and amphibians. Another is *Bacillus thuringiensis,* commonly called "Bt." It comes as a powder, which is actually a mixture of dried bacterial spores and crystals of the toxin they release. Bt kills mosquito larvae both by a direct toxic effect and by causing an overwhelming infection. It is no threat to mammals, birds, fish, or frogs, but there may be collateral damage to a wide range of insects, including beetles, butterflies, and moths.

Backyard "bug zappers" or more expensive machines purported to attract, trap, and kill mosquitoes have not been proven to significantly decrease exposure to mosquito bites. Theoretically, these devices could increase the number of mosquitoes in a given area, if they attract more efficiently than they kill. For the cost of some of these machines you might be able to purchase more than one hundred bottles of repellent.

In an era when many medical consumers are increasingly attracted to "natural" products and remedies, a substance called N,N-diethyl-3-methylbenzamide makes many consumers skeptical. However, this chemical, commonly known as DEET, remains the most effective insect repellant known, as proven by some recent research.

Drs. Mark Fradin and John Day of the Universities of North

TABLE 17.1
Efficacy of insect repellents

Product	Active ingredients	Minutes until first bite
OFF! Deep Woods	DEET 23.8%	301.5
Sawyer Controlled Release	DEET 20%	234.4
OFF! Skintastic	DEET 6.65%	112.4
Bite Blocker for Kids	Soybean oil 2%	94.6
OFF! Skintastic for Kids	DEET 4.75%	88.4
Skin-So-Soft Bug Guard Plus	IR3535 7.5%	22.9
Natrapel	Citronella 10%	19.7
Herbal Armor	Citronella 10%, peppermint oil 2.5%, cedar oil 2%, lemongrass oil 1%, geranium oil 0.05%	18.9
Green Ban for People	Citronella 10%; peppermint oil 2%	14.0
Buzz Away	Citronella 5%	13.5
Skin-So-Soft Bug Guard	Citronella 0.1%	10.3
Skin-So-Soft Bath Oil	Various oils, soaps, and scents	9.6
Skin-So-Soft Suncare	Citronella 0.05%	2.8
Gone Original Wristband	DEET 9.5%	0.3
Repello Wristband	DEET 9.5%	0.2
Gone Plus Repelling Wristband	Citronella 25%	0.2

SOURCE: Adapted with permission from Fradin, M. S., and Day, J. F. "Comparative Efficacy of Insect Repellents against Mosquito Bites." *New England Journal of Medicine* 347 (2002): 13–18.

Carolina and Florida conducted a very simple, yet carefully controlled experiment comparing a wide range of commercially available repellents. Volunteers positioned their arms, from the elbow to the fingertips, in a cage filled with hungry mosquitoes, then researchers observed until how much time elapsed until the very first bite occurred. The results are shown in table 17.1.

All concentrations of DEET are effective when applied to

the skin, with higher concentrations lasting longer. The impregnated wristbands do not deter mosquitoes because DEET's repellent effect extends only for four centimeters (1½ inches). Because it works by vaporizing from your skin, do not cover it up with sunscreen. When applying both sunscreen and repellent, apply sunscreen first. This way, the repellent will work just as well as if it were applied alone, but you may want to use a stronger strength of sunscreen. Sunscreen loses one-third of its protective effect when applied under DEET.

If you are successful at averting mosquito bites, you will almost certainly avoid West Nile fever and its complications. However, mosquito bites are not the only way the virus has been transmitted. In August 2002, a man died in a motor vehicle accident in the state of Georgia. As part of the effort to save him, numerous blood transfusions were administered. When he died, four of his organs were transplanted into four needy recipients. All four recipients developed West Nile fever. Subsequently, blood banks identified many persons who became infected after receiving blood transfusions infected with West Nile virus.

Now, organ donors are tested, blood donors answer screening questions, and blood banks test their blood for West Nile. Few of the 4.5 million persons who receive blood annually in the United States will become infected with the virus. However, as with HIV, rarely, an infected donor will slip by. One technique to avoid a whole range of infections is to only accept transfusions when there is no possible alternative.

Mad cow disease

Dr. Stanley B. Prusiner, an academic neurologist in San Francisco, won the Nobel Prize in Physiology or Medicine for 1997. Speaking at the Nobel Banquet on December 10, 1996, he said, "People often ask me why I persisted in doing research on a subject that was so controversial." His comments were an understatement.

Dr. Prusiner, the discoverer of an entirely new form of infectious agent—the prion—was pummeled by his scientific community and by the press for his theories. In an autobiography Prusiner wrote, "the personal attacks of the naysayers at times became very vicious." Prusiner first introduced the term "prion" in the spring of 1982. After that, he writes, "Publication of this manuscript . . . set off a firestorm. Virologists were generally incredulous." Prusiner had run up against a mountain of doubt because he described a radically new type of germ. This microbe had no DNA and no RNA—it was made up only of protein. He put the term "prion" together from "protein" and "infection."

When Dr. Prusiner was doing his early and groundbreaking work, he had no idea that prion diseases were about to emerge from obscurity. Originally, he worked with a rare sheep disorder called "scrapie" and rarer human disorders called "kuru" and "Creutzfeldt-Jakob disease." The first report of variant Creutzfeldt-Jakob disease came from the United Kingdom in 1996. This disease is frightening because it affects the brain of young persons; there is no treatment for it and it is uniformly fatal. There have been over 150 cases to date, almost all in persons who resided in the United Kingdom.

So far, only one typical case has occurred in the United States. In early November 2001, a twenty-two-year-old British girl saw a doctor in Florida for depression and memory loss. She had moved to Florida in 1992. Her symptoms were affecting her work and she was referred to a psychologist. In early December 2001, she received a traffic ticket for failing to yield the right of way. By mid-December her muscles began to twitch involuntarily. She was evaluated at a local emergency room where she was thought to be having panic attacks and was given an anti-anxiety medication. Soon after, though, she found she could not always walk straight, had difficulty dressing herself, and then lost bladder control. By the summer of 2002 she was bedridden, noncommunicative, and near death. Further tests (done on a biopsy of her tonsils) were positive for the prion that causes variant Creutzfeldt-Jakob disease.

This case is illustrative of the Creutzfeldt-Jakob "variant" because, before 1996, Creutzfeldt-Jakob disease occurred in old individuals and started out with muscular problems. This new variant has afflicted men and women who died at an average age of twenty-eight and initially experienced psychiatric symptoms. Although patients with this illness deteriorate rapidly, there is a very long delay—years or decades—from when prions enter their bodies to when the first symptoms start. Victims most likely ingested the prions in hamburgers.

Another prion disease, bovine spongiform encephalopathy (BSE)—commonly called "mad cow disease"—was raging in British cows just before the first case of variant Creutzfeldt-Jakob disease. The incidence of BSE peaked in 1993, when nearly one thousand cows a week were diagnosed with the disease. At that time, farmers in the United Kingdom would feed ground sheep parts to cattle and some of the sheep that were used as feed had scrapie. This allowed the prions to jump from one species to another.

Meatpackers gave prions a second opportunity to jump species, this time from cattle to humans. A cost-efficient method of harvesting beef from slaughtered cattle called "mechanically recovered meat" was to blame. This process, now banned in Europe, contaminated meat (which is the cow's muscle) with tissue stripped from the nervous system, where the highest concentrations of prions reside.

The prion protein that causes mad cow disease has been found in animals' brain, spinal cord, eye, and bone marrow. So, the best technique to avoid acquiring variant Creutzfeldt-Jakob is to vary what you eat. (Cooking may not inactivate

---

TABLE 17.2
Strategies to lower your risk of acquiring mad cow disease

For the risk averse:

❑ Eat only boneless beef
❑ Avoid chopped beef

For everyone:

❑ Do not eat brains

---

prions.) As the risk is very low—perhaps about one case per ten billion servings of beef in the United Kingdom—it is perfectly reasonable not to do anything to ameliorate that risk. There is now a slight degree of risk in North America as well, as BSE has been diagnosed in Canadian cows and on December 23, 2003, one cow in the state of Washington was diagnosed with it. The problem with assessing risk in the United States is that very little is done in the meatpacking industry to prevent and detect disease, so there could be more prions in our food supply than we know.

Not eating brain (some people do, usually as a brain sandwich!) is a reasonable first step to lower your risk of acquiring variant Creutzfeldt-Jakob disease. To eliminate your future risk you would need to become a vegetarian. Some vegetarian foods are prepared with beef substances (e.g. broth or gelatin), but to date no prions have been found in these substances. In between these two poles of risk aversion, one might decide to only eat steak (see table 17.2). Chopped beef may be more likely to become contaminated with errant beef parts. Also, an easy way you might lower your risk is limit your beef intake to fillets, not ribs, T-bones, or rib eye cuts, as prions may be found in bone marrow. Regardless of the approach you take, your risk from eating beef is very low to start with.

Beef, however, is not the only food Americans eat that may infect them with prions. As far back as the 1960s, many of our deer and elk have experienced their own prion-induced brain infection. This infection in wild game is called "chronic wasting disease." Three men in the upper Midwest who had participated in wild game feasts died of Creutzfeldt-Jakob disease, possibly a result of the wild game they ate. Two of them were from Wisconsin and one was from Minnesota.

Medical experts most carefully studied the man from Minnesota. He was fifty-five years old when he became ill and died. In May 1999 he reported three months of progressive difficulty in writing and difficulty walking. Brain scans were normal. In June 1999 he developed speech abnormalities, muscular twitching, and some dementia. Creutzfeldt-Jakob disease was diagnosed and proven at autopsy in July 1999. This man had eaten venison repeatedly and had participated in twelve wild game feasts held at a remote cabin in the Wisconsin woods.

Chronic wasting disease, so far, has been found in deer or elk in Colorado, Illinois, Kansas, Minnesota, Montana, Nebraska, New Mexico, Oklahoma, South Dakota, and Wisconsin. Until more is known, avoiding venison, at least from these areas, might be another strategy to lower one's risk of acquiring a prion disease.

Severe Acute Respiratory Syndrome (SARS)

For now, SARS is quiescent. However, you should consider it a sleeping giant. SARS is frightfully contagious and frequently lethal. When it broke out of Guangdong Province, China, in 2003, spreading mostly in Vietnam, Singapore, and Hong Kong, over 8,000 persons became ill and 774 deaths were recorded. The good news is that the world learned a lot about it very fast and we will be better prepared in the future.

SARS is a pneumonia, or lung infection. It is caused by a particular virus, the SARS-associated coronavirus, and is transmitted through the air from person to person. Most SARS patients had a clear history of exposure to other SARS patients or known SARS-affected area. If SARS visits us again, we will all hear about it. Public Health Departments maintain a keen watch.

The good news is that we know how to prevent SARS from spreading. Masks work. It was shown in China that among citizens, the use of masks was strongly protective from SARS. In Toronto and Hong Kong, it was those health care workers who failed to consistently cover their nose and mouth that succumbed to SARS. The thick, tight-fitting N-95 respirator mask is thought to be the best protection, but ordinary surgical masks work too.

If SARS returns, avoid high-transmission areas (particularly medical clinics) and cover your mouth and nose. These simple strategies have been shown to provide very effective protection.

18 *Bioterrorism*

Bob Stevens loved the outdoors. He enjoyed gardening. He loved to fish. According to friends, he would sometimes stop on the way from his home in Lantana, Florida, to work in Boca Raton and cast his line into a pond or canal. In early September 2001, Bob had no idea that a plot was unfolding in the air above him. Mohammed Atta, the kingpin of the September 11, 2001 attacks, and two of his accomplices were flight training at Palm Beach County Airport. This airport is less than one mile from the Stevenses' home. Forty miles to the west, in Belle Glade, the terrorists were making inquiries at a crop-dusting operation.

Bob Stevens became the first victim to die from inhalation anthrax in 2001. However, his illness was no fluke of nature. Anthrax, a bacterial infection caused by *Bacillus anthracis*, does not occur naturally in the United States. Rather, Mr. Stevens, who became ill on September 30 and died on October 5, was the victim of bioterrorism.

Although there was early speculation that Bob Stevens had inhaled anthrax spores dropped from the sky by members of al Qaeda, it later became clear that the disease arrived at Mr. Stevens's workplace by mail. Sending anthrax through the mail is an effective form of bioterrorism because the intent is to attract a lot of attention and stir fear. To be a successful bioterrorist, you need only to infect a few individuals. Fortunately, however, this is not so easily done. Although anthrax remains the most workable agent among the choices available, it is not easy to spread. If al Qaeda, or others, had tried to disseminate anthrax spores more widely, they failed. There are many technical problems that any would-be bioterrorist would have to overcome to successfully use anthrax as a weapon. I choose not to enumerate these obstacles lest I provide a guidebook for criminals.

Although someone was lethally successful eleven times in 2001, terrorists have tried before to use anthrax as a weapon and failed. One such group, Aum Shinrikyo, responsible for the release of sarin nerve gas in a Tokyo subway in 1995, had dispersed aerosols of anthrax (and botulism) throughout Tokyo on at least eight previous occasions. None of these attacks succeeded in producing illness.

In addition to the intricacies required to spread anthrax, we have some excellent tools to foil would-be assailants: a vaccine and a host of antibiotics. Anthrax vaccine is an inactivated vaccine, that is, it contains no living organisms. It was licensed in 1970, so there is a good bit of experience with it. It is given as a six-dose series and is mandated for all U.S. military active- and reserve-duty personnel. It becomes protective after the second dose and no serious adverse effects have been related to the vaccine. (Local injection site and minor systemic reactions such as muscle aches occur temporarily in 10–20 percent of those vaccinated.) More anthrax vaccine is being produced so that it is available to civilians at risk in the event of future attacks. Better anthrax vaccines (fewer shots, longer immunity) are in development.

Four drugs that are approved by the Food and Drug Administration are likely to prevent anthrax following exposure: ciprofloxacin, gatifloxacin, moxifloxacin, and doxycycline. This use of antibiotics (called chemoprophylaxis) is indicated only after a known exposure and should be continued for sixty days. In the event of an attack, our Public Health Service would make antibiotics available to those who need it. This program is called the National Pharmaceutical Stockpile Program and is managed by the Centers for Disease Control and Prevention.

The U.S. government is also doing what it can to detect another attack as soon as possible. One way it is approaching this is by setting up a network of detectors that are extremely sensitive to minute amounts of anthrax or other pathogens' DNA in air samples. Known as the BioWatch system, it is managed by the Department of Homeland Security. About a dozen sites in each of thirty-one cities across the country have the detectors, but the list of pathogens and the location of the devices are, naturally, secret.

If another anthrax attack escapes detection, and we are robbed of the opportunity to take preventive steps, an unvaccinated individual exposed by inhalation would experience the following symptoms: After an incubation period of about one week, a flulike syndrome develops. There may be fever, nausea, muscle aches, and cough. During this prodromal phase anthrax is treatable with antibiotics but is very difficult to diagnose. Only a chest x-ray, if characteristic, would allow a doctor to pick it up. If untreated, after just another day or two, the victim becomes seriously ill. Meningitis, respiratory failure, and shock commonly occur. Antibiotics are of little help at this stage.

As we all know, anthrax can be a killer. But there are many other agents that present potentially lethal bioterrorist threats. Each would pose its own set of difficulties for a perpetrator.

Plague is probably the next most likely infectious disease a terrorist might try to use. Plague is a bacterial infection caused by *Yersinia pestis*. If it were dispersed in an aerosol, it would cause a pneumonia or "pneumonic plague"—the most deadly form. After an incubation period of only two to three days, a victim would experience the sudden onset of malaise, fever, chills, headache, cough, and bloody sputum. Treatment with antibiotics can be effective, but only if begun within the first twenty-four hours of illness. A vaccine for plague is not currently available. Unlike anthrax, plague pneumonia can be spread from person to person, as it was during the great "Black Death" epidemic in Europe in the fourteenth century. Secondary cases could arise following an initial plague attack.

Despite high publicity, smallpox would be one of the least likely agents for a successful terrorist attack. Whereas anthrax and plague bacteria can be gathered from animals in the environment, the smallpox virus, *variola*, only infects humans. The last naturally occurring case of smallpox was in 1979 and smallpox stockpiles are maintained only in laboratories in Atlanta and in Novosibirsk, Russia. However, there is no way to verify whether other nations secretly retained the virus, and some have questioned the integrity of the Russian stockpile. So, although there are no data to suggest that any smallpox virus is available to wrongdoers, many are concerned about such a possibility.

Smallpox would challenge terrorists with even more difficulties (which, again, I prefer not to discuss) than the bacterial agents. One of these difficulties is that some Americans are immune to smallpox. Many of us would like to know our status. If you were vaccinated twice, you are immune. Persons who were vaccinated twice usually are individuals who received a routine childhood vaccination, given until 1972, and then were given a booster before travel. If you were vaccinated once and have a visible scar on your arm, you may have at least partial immunity for as long as seventy-five years after the vaccine was given.

The current smallpox vaccine is a variant of the first vaccine ever invented (Jenner, 1796). This vaccine is widely expected to be protective even if given as long as four days after exposure. A new vaccine is under development. It is likely to be more effective and a lot less risky. Furthermore, some of our newest antiviral antibiotics may be effective against smallpox.

The viral hemorrhagic fevers (Ebola, Marburg, and Lassa fever among them) are all contagious and deadly, but highly technical to work with and even more problematic to dissemi-nate. These infections, botulism, and tularemia complete the list of the most likely infections a terrorist might spread (see table 18.1). Unfortunately, there are many more candidate agents and the next attack might be unforeseen.

Bioterrorism and biological warfare are not new. They have a long past and there is no reason to think they will not occur in the future. In medieval times, armies catapulted cadavers with plague and typhus over the fortress walls of their enemy. During the French and Indian War in the American colonies, British forces gave contaminated blankets from hospitals to Na-tive Americans to disseminate smallpox. During World War I, Germany exported sheep they had infected with the bacterial disease meliodosis. In World War II, Japan experimented widely in Asia with anthrax and plague. Toward the end of the cold war, the accidental release from an anthrax plant in Sverdlovsk, Russia, killed sixty-eight infected civilians. It would be naïve to think that further biological attacks are not in our future.

While we have the most successful and sophisticated pub-lic health system that has ever existed, we are not by any means fully protected from bioterrorism. Nor can we be completely protected from food borne illnesses, HIV, TB, respiratory viruses, and many other germs in search of opportunities to invade. It is vital that we all learn how to take precautions and protect ourselves.

TABLE 18.1
Highest potential bioterrorism risks

Disease	Main symptoms	Treatment	Protection
Inhalation anthrax	Flulike at first Chest pain, shortness of breath, headache, nausea, diarrhea	Clindamycin Ciprofloxacin	Various antibiotics Vaccine (Not transmitted from person to person)
Pneumonic plague	High fever, cough (usually bloody), shortness of breath	Doxycycline Gentamicin	Masks Early treatment
Smallpox	Fever, back pain, vomiting, headache with rash 2–3 days later Pox most abundant on face	Cidofovir might work	Masks Vaccine Immune globulin
Botulism	Weakness, drooping eyelids, double vision, slurred speech	Antitoxin	Avoid contaminated foods Boil or intensely heat suspect foods
Tularemia	Fever, headache, chest pain, dry cough, conjunctivitis	Gentamicin Doxycycline	Early antibiotic treatment Vaccine only experimental (Not transmitted from person to person)
Viral hemorrhagic fevers (e.g., Ebola)	Fever, severe headache, muscle pain Rash and bleeding around the fifth day	Intravenous fluids and blood transfusions Ribavirin may work for some species, but not Ebola	Strict isolation of victims with masks, gloves, gowns and incineration of patients' waste and supplies

Vaccination schedules

Recommended childhood immunizations

At birth:

hepatitis B

At 2 months:

hepatitis B
diphtheria-tetanus-pertussis (DTP)
inactivated poliovirus vaccine (IPV)
Hemophilus influenzae type B (Hib)
pneumococcal conjugate vaccine (Prevnar)

At 4 months:

diphtheria-tetanus-pertussis (DTP)
inactivated poliovirus vaccine (IPV)
Hemophilus influenzae type B (Hib)
pneumococcal conjugate vaccine (Prevnar)

At 6 months:

hepatitis B
diphtheria-tetanus-pertussis (DTP)
inactivated poliovirus vaccine (IPV)
pneumococcal conjugate vaccine (Prevnar)
influenza vaccine (yearly until age 2)

At 12 months:

diphtheria-tetanus-pertussis (DTP)
Hemophilus influenzae type B (Hib)
measles-mumps-rubella (MMR)
varicella (Varivax)
pneumococcal conjugate vaccine (Prevnar)

At 4 to 6 years:

diphtheria-tetanus-pertussis (DTP)
oral polio vaccine (OPV)
measles-mumps-rubella (MMR)

Adult immunizations

❑ *Vaccine's nickname:* BCG.

❑ *Real name:* Bacille Calmette-Guérin.

Expected benefit: Can sometimes diminish your risk of getting TB (see chapter 9).
Dosing schedule: 1 dose.

Boosters: Not recommended.

Who should get it: As discussed in chapter 9.

Side effects:* A live vaccine, not to be taken by those without intact immune systems. May turn your PPD skin test positive.

❑ *Vaccine's nickname:* Chickenpox vaccine.

❑ *Real name:* Varicella virus vaccine live (Oka/Merck) (Varivax).

Expected benefit: It will substantially diminish the risk of getting chickenpox if you've never had it and become exposed; if you get chickenpox anyway, it will be mild.

Dosing schedule: Over 13 years old, two doses, 4 to 8 weeks apart.

Boosters: Unknown, but not before 8 years.

Who should get it: Adolescents and adults who have never had chickenpox and work with small children, are in contact with others whose immune systems are poor, are women of child-bearing age (but not pregnant), or have been exposed to chickenpox in the prior three days.

Side effects:* Pain and redness at the injection site (25 percent), a fever (10 percent), or a mild chickenpoxlike rash (5 percent).

❑ *Vaccine's nickname:* Flu shot.

❑ *Real name:* Inactivated whole and split influenza virus vaccine.

Expected benefit: Diminishes your chance of getting influenza, and thereby, of pneumonia. Effectiveness varies from year to year.

Dosing schedule: A single yearly injection, usually around the 1st of November.

Boosters: None; a new vaccine is made yearly.

Who should get it: Everyone over 65, all medical personnel, and others at high risk for respiratory infection (see chapter 8).

*Side effects:** A third of recipients have a sore arm; fewer get a low-grade fever and muscle aches.

❑   *Vaccine's nickname:* German measles vaccine.

❑   *Real name:* Live, attenuated rubella vaccine.

Expected benefit: You won't get rubella if you've received this vaccine. More importantly, you won't give birth to a child with congenital defects caused by rubella.

Dosing schedule: 1 dose, given in the MMR vaccination for measles, mumps, and rubella. For women of childbearing potential, take only during menses.

Boosters: None.

Who should get it: Everyone, as part of childhood vaccination series. Immunity is often checked when applying for a marriage license, when contemplating pregnancy, or when working in a hospital. Get vaccinated if testing shows you're not immune.

*Side effects:** If you are female and not immune, you might get transient arthritis and rash.

❑   *Vaccine's nickname:* Hepatitis A vaccine.

❑   *Real name:* Hepatitis A vaccine, inactivated (Havrix).

Expected benefit: You will become immune to hepatitis A infection beginning 2 weeks after vaccination.

Dosing schedule: Over age 18, a single dose. Children receive 2 doses a month apart.

Boosters: A booster after 6 to 12 months will make the vaccine's effect long lasting.

Who should get it: Travelers to underdeveloped nations; Native Americans; persons exposed to hepatitis A (with globulin given simultaneously); those in a community in which there's a hepatitis A outbreak.

*Side effects:** No more than a sore arm.

❑ *Vaccine's nickname:* Hepatitis B vaccine.

❑ *Real name:* Recombinant hepatitis B surface antigen.

Expected benefit: Excellent protection against hepatitis B.

Dosing schedule: Must be given in the arm. Three shots—repeats at 1 and 6 months after initial injection.

Boosters: No standard recommendation, but good for 10 years in persons whose immune status is intact.

Who should get it: Medical care workers; persons residing for more than 6 months in places where hepatitis B is common (for example, Africa and Asia); persons living with a carrier; and others (also see chapter 11).

*Side effects:** Soreness at the site of injection.

❑ *Vaccine's nickname:* Hib.

❑ *Real name:* *Hemophilus influenzae* type b conjugate (Hib).

Expected benefit: Prevents a bacterial infection that can cause meningitis and pneumonia, more commonly in children than in adults.

Dosing schedule: 1 dose.

Boosters: Not recommended.

Who should get it: Anyone whose spleen in absent or diseased (see chapter 13).

*Side effects:** Mild local reactions in 10 percent of persons vaccinated.

❑ *Vaccine's nickname:* Japanese encephalitis vaccine.

❑ *Real name:* Inactivated Japanese B encephalitis vaccine.

Expected benefit: Prevents this infection of the nervous system.

Dosing schedule: 3 doses a week apart.

Boosters: In 2 years.

Who should get it: Those who will be residing in rural Asia.

*Side effects:** Mild reactions at the site of injection.

❑ *Vaccine's nickname:* Measles shot.

❑ *Real name:* Live, attenuated measles vaccine; usually as MMR combination for measles, mumps, and rubella.

Expected benefit: If your MMR vaccination is up to date, you won't get measles (rubeola).

Dosing schedule: For previously vaccinated adults, one dose.

Boosters: None (after a lifetime total of 2 doses are received).

Who should get it: People born after 1956 who never had measles and who only had a single prior measles vaccine.

*Side effects:** A live vaccine—not for immune-compromised individuals; made in eggs—not for those who are allergic; it can occasionally cause transient fever and rash.

❑ *Vaccine's nickname:* Meningitis vaccine.

❑ *Real name:* Tetravalent meningococcal polysaccharide vaccine.

Expected benefit: Bacterial meningitis from 4 of the most common strains becomes very unlikely.

Dosing schedule: 1 dose.

Boosters: About every 3 years.

Who should get it: Travelers to areas where meningitis is frequent (see chapter 7), people whose spleen has been removed or malfunctions, and, sometimes, large groups of people during an epidemic.

*Side effects:** Mild local reactions only.

❑ *Vaccine's nickname:* Mumps shot.

❑ *Real name:* Live, attenuated mumps vaccine; part of MMR (see German measles vaccine and Measles shot).

Expected benefit: Prevents you from getting mumps.

Dosing schedule: 1 dose, given along with measles and rubella in MMR vaccination.

Boosters: None.

Who should get it: Given routinely as part of the childhood series.

*Side effects:** Minimal.

❑ *Vaccine's nickname:* Pneumonia shot.

❑ *Real name:* pneumococcal polysaccharide vaccine (Pneumovax-23).

Expected benefit: Diminishes your risk of developing common pneumonia.

Dosing schedule: 1 dose.

Boosters: Persons with kidney disease, sickle cell disease, and some others may want to get a booster injection in 6 years.

Who should get it: All over 65 and many others (see chapter 8).

Side effects:* Half the recipients get redness and pain in the arm after the shot, but fever and a flulike reaction occur in 1 percent.

❑ *Vaccine's nickname:* Polio shot.

❑ *Real name:* Enhanced potency trivalent poliovirus vaccine, inactivated (IPV).

Expected benefit: If your polio vaccine is up to date, you won't get polio.

Dosing schedule: The primary series is given in childhood. The booster is a single injection.

Boosters: Only one, if needed.

Who should get it: Anyone traveling to underdeveloped nations (see chapter 7).

Side effects:* Minimal.

❑ *Vaccine's nickname:* Rabies shots.

❑ *Real name:* Human diploid cell rabies vaccine (HDCV).

Expected benefit: Prevents rabies in those who have been exposed or those likely to be. To be reliable after a bite, rabies immune globulin must also be given.

Dosing schedule: Postexposure, 1 shot in the arm on days 0, 3, 7, 14, and 28. Globulin (usually 2 injections in the buttock) is given also on day 0. Preexposure, 3 doses in the arm on days 0, 7, and 28; if later exposed, 2 more doses are given.

Boosters: About every 2 years.

Who should get it: Anyone who may have been exposed to rabies (see appendix C). Preexposure vaccination is for anyone traveling for longer than 1 month to areas where rabies is a constant threat, and for animal handlers.

Side effects:* 25 percent of recipients get local reactions, fewer get nausea and headache; nervous system reactions occur rarely. Boosters can cause allergic reactions like hives.

❑ *Vaccine's nickname:* Tetanus shot.

❑ *Real name:* Diphtheria-tetanus toxoid (Td).

Expected benefit: You will not get either disease if your Td vaccination is up to date.

Dosing schedule: The initial series is given in childhood.

Boosters: Every 10 years. If you are traveling abroad or have a deep or dirty wound, then every 5 years.

Who should get it: Everyone.

Side effects:* Sore arm and occasionally a flulike illness for a day or two. Allergy is rare.

❑ *Vaccine's nickname:* Typhoid pills.

❑ *Real name:* Typhoid vaccine, oral (Ty21a, oral).

Expected benefit: Cuts your risk of catching typhoid fever by 79 to 90 percent.

Dosing schedule: 1 pill every other day for 4 doses. Refrigerate.

Boosters: Every 5 years.

Who should get it: Travelers to underdeveloped nations who are going off usual tourist routes.

Side effects:* This is a live vaccine, not to be taken by immune-deficient persons. If you are taking antibiotics, it won't work. It can sometimes give you nausea and diarrhea.

❑ *Vaccine's nickname:* Typhoid shot.

❑ *Real name:* Vi capsular polsaccharide typhoid vaccine (Typhim Vi).

Expected benefit: Cuts your risk of typhoid fever by about 75 percent.

Dosing schedule: A single injection.

Boosters: Every 2 years.

Who should get it: Travelers to underdeveloped nations who are going off usual tourist routes.

*Side effects:** You might get a sore, red arm; 7 percent of the time the sore area is more than a half-inch wide.

*None of these vaccines should be taken routinely by pregnant women. Some—for example, rabies vaccine—may occasionally become necessary. Vaccines are usually not given to any person who has reacted severely or had an allergy to a previous dose. Some vaccines contain small amounts of egg or certain antibiotics; be sure to list your allergies for the nurse before receiving vaccine.

Antibiotics to prevent infective endocarditis

For dental, oral, or upper respiratory tract procedures in patients who are at risk: amoxicillin 2.0 grams (usually in 4 pills) by mouth 1 hour before the procedure, then half that dose 6 hours later. If allergic to penicillin, substitute clindamycin (Cleocin), 600 mg prior and 300 mg after.

For high-risk persons and those unable to take oral medications: ampicillin 2 grams intravenously 30 minutes before the procedure and then 1.0 grams intravenously or intramuscularly, or amoxicillin 1.5 gm by mouth 6 hours later. If allergic to penicillin, substitute clindamycin (Cleocin), 600 mg intravenously 30 minutes prior to the procedure and again intravenously or by mouth 6 hours later.

For genitourinary (urologic) or gastrointestinal procedures: ampicillin 2 grams, plus gentamicin 1.5 mg/kg intravenously 30 minutes before the procedure; repeat 8 hours later, or just give amoxicillin 1.5 grams by mouth. If allergic to penicillin, 1.0 grams of vancomycin intravenously replaces ampicillin and amoxicillin.

NOTE: There are many reason why your physician, knowing your unique situation, may want you to veer from these recommendations.

SOURCES: Adapted from A. S. Dejani, A. L. Bisno, K. J. Chung, D. T. Durack, M. Freed, M. A. Gerber, A. W. Karchmer, H. D. Millard, S. Rahimtoola, S. T. Shulman, C. Watanakunakorn, and K. A. Taubert, "Prevention of Bacterial Endocarditis: Recommendations by the American Heart Association," *Journal of the American Medical Association* 264 (1990): 2919.

APPENDIX C *Rabies*

Rabies handled correctly is always preventable. Rabies allowed to cause disease is always fatal. After the bite of an animal suspected to be rabid, clean the wound immediately with soap and water, and get specific treatment—with both rabies immune globulin and rabies vaccine—within 24 hours. If for any reason there is a delay, better late than never. Nonbite exposure is when your mouth, eye, or any wound gets contaminated with an animal's secretions. Although not as risky as a bite, the same preventive treatment is needed.

Animal	Start rabies shots immediately?	Ultimately consider animal rabid and finish the series?
Vaccinated dog or cat behaving normally.	No	No
Unvaccinated dog or cat behaving normally.	No	Decide based on 10 days of of observation by a veterinarian.
Dog or cat behaving abnormally, especially if attack was unprovoked.	Yes	Yes, if the Public Health Service tells you there's rabies in your area; the animal may need to be sacrificed and examined.
Dog or cat that runs away after biting and cannot be found.	Yes	Yes, if the Public Health Service tells you there's rabies in your area.
Fox, skunk, racoon, bat, woodchuck, or other carnivore.	Yes	Yes, unless the animal is sacrificed, its brain is examined for rabies particles, and the finding is negative.
Livestock.	No	You must ask the veterinarian.
Rabbit, hare, squirrel, rat, or mouse.	No	No, unless the animal's brain is examined for rabies particles and is positive.

SOURCES: Adapted from the CDC publication "Rabies Prevention—United States, 1991: Recommendations of the Immunization Practices Advisory Committee (ACIP)," *Morbidity and Mortality Weekly Report* 40, RR-3 (1991): 1.

Bibliography

Introduction

Smith, J. S., Fishbein, D. B., Rupprecht, C. E., and Clark, K. "Unexplained Rabies in Three Immigrants in the United States: A Virologic Investigation." *New England Journal of Medicine* 324 (1991): 205–211.

1 The common cold

Garibaldi, R. A. "Epidemiology of Community-Acquired Respiratory Tract Infections in Adults." *American Journal of Medicine* 78, Supp. 6B (1985): 32.

Gwaltney, J. M. "Rhinovirus." In *The Principles and Practice of Infectious Disease*, 4th ed., edited by G. L. Mandell, J. E. Bennett, and R. G. Douglas. New York: Wiley, 1994, p. 1656.

Myrvik, Q. N. "Immunology and Nutrition." In *Modern Nutrition in Health and Disease*, 8th ed., edited by M. E. Shils, J. A. Olson, and M. Shike. Philadelphia: Lea and Febiger, 1994, p. 652.

2 Strep throat and other strep infections

Bisno, A. L. "Group A Streptococcal Infections and Acute Rheumatic Fever." *New England Journal of Medicine* 325 (1991): 783.

Centers for Disease Control. "Invasive Group A Streptococcal Infections—United Kingdom, 1994." *Morbidity and Mortality Weekly Report* 43 (1994): 401.

Dajani, A. S., Bisno, A. K., Chung, K. J., Durack, D. T., Gerber, M. A., Kaplan, E. L., Millard, H. D., Randolph, M. F., Shulman, S. T., and Watanakunakorn, C. "Prevention of Rheumatic Fever." *Circulation* 78 (1988): 1082.

Demers, B., Simor, A. E., Vellend, H., Schlievert, P. M., Byrne, S., Jamieson, F., Walmsley, S., and Low, D. E. "Severe Invasive Group A Streptococcal Infections in Ontario, Canada: 1987–1991." *Clinical Infectious Diseases* 16 (1993): 792.

Randall, D. A., Parker, G. S., and Kennedy, K. S. "Indications for Tonsillectomy and Adenoidectomy." *American Family Physician* 44 (1991): 1639.

Schwartz, B., Elliott, J. A., Butler, J. C., Simon, P. A., Jameson, B. L., Welch, G. E., and Facklam, R. R. "Clusters of Invasive Group A Streptococcal Infections in Family, Hospital, and Nursing Home Settings." *Clinical Infectious Diseases* 15 (1992): 277.

Stromberg, A., Romanus, V., and Burman, L. G. "Outbreak of Group A Streptococcal Bacteremia in Sweden: An Epidemiologic and Clinical Study." *Journal of Infectious Diseases* 164 (1991): 595.

Tanz, R. R., Shulman, S. T., Barthel, M. J., Willert, C., and Yogev, R. "Penicillin Plus Rifampin Eradicates Pharyngeal Carriage of Group A Streptococci." *Journal of Pediatrics* 106 (1985): 876.

3 Urinary tract infections

Avorn, J., Monane, M., Gurwitz, J. H., Glynn, R. J., Choodnovskiy, I., and Lipsitz, L. A. "Reduction of Bacteriuria and Pyuria after Ingestion of Cranberry Juice." *Journal of the American Medical Association* 271 (1994): 751.

Foxman, B., and Frerichs, R. R. "Epidemiology of Urinary Tract Infection: Diaphragm Use and Sexual Intercourse." *American Journal of Public Health* 75 (1985): 1308.

Hooton, T. M., Hillier, S., Johnson, C., Roberts, P. L., and Stamm, W. E. "*Escherichia coli* Bacteriuria and Contraceptive Method." *Journal of the American Medical Association* 265 (1991): 64.

Pfau, A., and Sacks, T. G. "Effective Postcoital Quinolone Prophylaxis of Recurrent Urinary Tract Infections in Women." *Journal of Urology* 152 (1994): 136.

Raz, R., and Stamm, W. E. "A Controlled Trial of Intravaginal Estriol in Postmenopausal Women with Recurrent Urinary Tract Infections." *New England Journal of Medicine* 329 (1993): 753.

Ronald, A. R., and Pattullo, A.L.S. "The Natural History of Urinary Infection in Adults." *Medical Clinics of North America* 75 (1991): 299.

Stapleton, A., Latham, R. H., Johnson, C., and Stamm, W. E. "Postcoital Antimicrobial Prophylaxis for Recurrent Urinary Tract Infection: A Randomized, Double-Blind, Placebo-Controlled Trial." *Journal of the American Medical Asociation* 264 (1990): 703.

Strom, B. L., Collins, M., West, S. L., Kreisberg, J., and Weller, S. "Sexual Activity, Contraceptive Use, and Other Risk Factors for Symptomatic and Asymptomatic Bacteriuria." *Annals of Internal Medicine* 107 (1987): 816.

4 Infections of the skin

Abersfeld, D. M., and Thomas, I. "Cutaneous Herpes Simplex Virus Infections." *American Family Physician* 43 (1991): 1655.

American Academy of Pediatrics Committee on Infectious Diseases. "Varicella Vaccine Update." *Pediatrics* 105 (2000): 136–141.

Anderson, N. J. "Cutaneous Dermatophytic Infections." *Postgraduate Medicine,* Special Report: Mycology, Forum II (1995): 14–17.

Bergus, G. R., and Johnson, J. S. "Superficial Tinea Infections." *American Family Physician* 48 (1993): 259.

Canoso, J. J., and Barza, M. "Soft Tissue Infections." *Rheumatic Disease Clinics of North America* 19 (1993): 293.

Hacker, S. M. "Common Infections of the Skin." *Postgraduate Medicine* 96 (1994): 43.

Kahm, R. M., and Goldstein, E.J.C. "Common Bacterial Skin Infections." *Postgraduate Medicine* 93 (1993): 175.

Sawyer, M. H., Chamberlin, C. J., Wu, Y. N., Aintablain, N., and Wallace, M. R. "Dectection of Varicella-Zoster Virus DNA in Air Samples from Hospital Rooms." *Journal of Infectious Diseases* 169 (1994): 91–94.

Stoeckle, M. Y., and Douglas, R. G. "Infectious Diseases." *Journal of the American Medical Association* 271 (1994): 1677.

5 *Lyme disease and tickborne infections*

Centers for Disease Control. "Lyme Disease—United States, 1993." *Morbidity and Mortality Weekly Report* 43 (1994): 564.

Centers for Disease Control and Prevention. "Final 2002 Reports of Notifiable Diseases." *Morbidity and Mortality Weekly Report* 52 (2003): 741–750.

Ginsberg, H., ed. *The Ecology and Environmental Management of Lyme Disease.* New Brunswick, N.J.: Rutgers University Press, 1993.

Fishbein, D. B., Dawson, J. E., and Robinson, L. E. "Human Ehrlichiosis in the United States, 1985 to 1990." *Annals of Internal Medicine* 120 (1994): 736.

Magid, D., Schwartz, B., Craft, J., and Schwartz, J. S. "Prevention of Lyme Disease after Tick Bites: A Cost-Effective Analysis." *New England Journal of Medicine* 327 (1992): 534.

Markowitz, L. E., Steere, A. C., Benach, J. L., Slade, J. D., and Broome, C. V. "Lyme Disease During Pregnancy." *Journal of the American Medical Association* 255 (1986): 3394.

Matuschka, F., and Spielman, A. "Images in Clinical Medicine: The Vector of the Lyme Disease Spirochete." *New England Journal of Medicine* 327 (1992): 542.

Needham, G. R. "Evaluation of Five Popular Methods for Tick Removal." *Pediatrics* 75 (1985): 997.

Steere, A. C. "Lyme Disease." *New England Journal of Medicine* 321 (1989): 586.

6 *Food poisoning*

Bartlett, J. G. "Antibiotic-Associated Diarrhea." *Clinical Infectious Diseases* 15 (1992): 573.

Bishai, W. R., and Sears, C. L. "Food Poisoning Syndromes." *Gastroenterology Clinics of North America* 22 (1993): 579.

Centers for Disease Control. "Multistate Outbreak of Viral Gastroenteritis Related to Consumption of Oysters: Louisiana, Maryland, Mississippi, and North Carolina, 1993." *Morbidity and Mortality Weekly Report* 42 (1993): 945.

Centers for Disease Control. "Foodborne Outbreaks of Enterotoxigenic *Escherichia coli:* Rhode Island and New Hampshire, 1993." *Morbidity and Mortality Weekly Report* 43 (1994): 81.

Centers for Disease Control and Prevention. "Preliminary FoodNet Data on the Incidence of Foodborne Illnesses—Selected Sites, United States, 2002." *Morbidity and Mortality Weekly Report* 52 (2003): 340–343.

Ching-Lee, M. R., Katz, A. R., Sasaki, D. M., Minette, H. P. "Salmonella Egg Survey in Hawaii: Evidence for Routine Bacterial Surveillance." *American Journal of Public Health* 81 (1991): 764–766.

Eastaugh, J., and Shepard, S. "Infectious and Toxic Syndromes from Fish and Shellfish Consumption." *Archives of Internal Medicine* 149 (1989): 1735.

Educational Foundation of the National Restaurant Association. *Applied Food Service Sanitation.* 4th ed. New York: Wiley, 1992.

Fang, G., Araujo, V., and Guerrant, R. L. "Enteric Infections Associated with

Exposure to Animals or Animal Products." *Infectious Disease Clinics of North America* 5 (1991): 681.

Hedberg, C. W., MacDonald, K. L., and Osterholm, M. T. "Changing Epidemiology of Foodborne Disease: A Minnesota Perspective." *Clinical Infectious Disease* 19 (1994): 671.

Humphrey, T. J., Greenwood, M., Gilbert, R. J., Rowe, B., and Chapman, P. A. "The Survival of Salmonellas in Shell Eggs Cooked under Simulated Domestic Conditions." *Epidemiology and Infection* 103 (1989): 35.

Irwin, K., Ballard, J., Grendon, J., and Kobayashi, J. "Results of Routine Restaurant Inspections Can Predict Outbreaks of Foodborne Illness: The Seattle–King County Experience." *American Journal of Public Health* 79 (1989): 586.

Jones, F. T., Rives, D. V., Carey, J. B. "Salmonella Contamination in Commercial Eggs and an Egg Production Facility." *Poultry Science* 743 (1995): 753–757.

Kelly, C. P., Pothoulakis, C., and LaMont, J. T. "*Clostridium Dificile* Colitis." *New England Journal of Medicine* 330 (1994): 257.

MacKenzie, W. R., Hoxie, N. J., Proctor, M. E., Gradus, M. S., Blair, K. A., Peterson, D. E., Kamierczak, J. J., Addiss, D. G., Fox, K. R., Rose, J. B., and Davis, J. P. "A Massive Outbreak in Milwaukee of Cryptosporidium Infection Transmitted through the Public Water Supply." *New England Journal of Medicine* 331 (1994): 161–167.

Mishu, B., Koehler, J., Lee, L. A., Rodrigue, D., Brenner, F. H., Blake, P., and Tauxe, R. V. "Outbreaks of *Salmonella enteritidis* Infections in the United States, 1985–1991." *Journal of Infectious Diseases* 169 (1994): 547.

Ongerth, J. E., Johnson, R. L., Macdonald, S. C., Frost, F., and Stibbs, H. H. "Backcountry Water Treatment to Prevent Giardiasis." *American Journal of Public Health* 79 (1989): 1633.

Schantz, P. M., Moore, A. C., Munoz, J. L., Hartman, B. J., Schaefer, J. A., Aron, A. M., Persaud, D., Sarti, E., Wilson, M., and Flisser, A. "Neurocysticercosis in an Orthodox Jewish Community in New York City." *New England Journal of Medicine* 327 (1992): 692.

Weber, J. T., Levine, W. C., Hopkins, D. P., and Tauxe, R. V. "Cholera in the United States, 1965–1991: Risks at Home and Abroad." *Archives of Internal Medicine* 154 (1994): 551.

7   Health hazards of travel

Cahill, T. "My Malaria." *Outside*, March 1994, pp. 90ff.

Centers for Disease Control. "Acute Schistosomiasis with Transverse Myelitis in American Students Returning from Kenya." *Morbidity and Mortality Weekly Report* 33 (1984): 445.

Centers for Disease Control. "Cholera Associated with International Travel, 1992." *Morbidity and Mortality Weekly Report* 41 (1992): 664.

Centers for Disease Control. *Health Information for International Travel, 1993.* Atlanta, Ga.: U.S. Department of Health and Human Services, 1993.

Ericsson, C. D., and DuPont, H. L. "Traveler's Diarrhea: Approaches to Prevention and Treatment." *Clinical Infectious Diseases* 16 (1993): 616.

Gottschalk, E. C., Jr. "Tour Your Insurance before Packing for a Trip." *Wall Street Journal*, January 31, 1994, p. C1.

Jelinek, T., Maiwald, H., Nothdurft, H. D., and Loscher, T. "Cutaneous Larva Migrans in Travelers: Synopsis of Histories, Symptoms, and Treatment in 98 Patients." *Clinical Infectious Diseases* 19 (1994): 1062.

Lobel, H. O., Phillips-Howard, P. A., Brandling-Bennett, A. D., Steffen, R., Campbell, C. C., Huong, A. Y., Were, J. B., and Moser, R. "Malaria Incidence and Prevention among European and North American Travelers to Kenya." *Bulletin of the World Health Organization* 68 (1990): 209.

Oldfield, E. C., Wallace, M. R., Hyams, K. C., Yousif, A. A., Lewis, D. E., and Bourgeios, A. L. "Endemic Infectious Diseases of the Middle East." *Clinical Infectious Diseases* 3, Supp. 3 (1991): S199.

"Typhoid Vaccination: Weighing the Options." *The Lancet* 340 (1992): 341 (editorial).

Woodruff, B. A., Pavia, T., and Blake, P. A. "A New Look at Typhoid Vaccination: Information for the Practicing Physician." *Journal of the American Medical Association* 265 (1991): 756.

Wyler, D. J. "Malaria Chemoprophylaxis for the Traveler." *New England Journal of Medicine* 329 (1993): 31.

8 Pneumonia and Legionnaires' disease

Centers for Disease Control. "Prevention and Control of Influenza: Recommendations of the Advisory Committee on Immunization Practices." *Morbidity and Mortality Weekly Report* 42, RR-6 (1993): 1.

Chapman, L. E., Tipple, M. A., Folger, S. G., Harmon, M., Kendal, A. P., Cox, N. J., and Schonberger, L. B. "Influenza: United States, 1988–89." *Morbidity and Mortality Weekly Report* 42, 22-1 (1992): 9.

Edelstein, P. H. "Legionnaires' Disease." *Clinical Infectious Diseases* 16 (1993): 741.

Paz, H. L., and Wood, C. A. "Pneumonia and Chronic Obstructive Disease." *Postgraduate Medicine* 90 (1991): 77.

9 Tuberculosis

Centers for Disease Control. "The Use of Preventive Therapy for Tuberculosis Infection in the United States: Recommendations of the Advisory Committee for Elimination of Tuberculosis." *Morbidity and Mortality Weekly Report* 39, RR-8 (1990): 9–12.

Dooley, S. W., Jarvis, W. R., Martone, W. J., and Snider, D. E., Jr. "Multidrug-Resistant Tuberculosis." *Annals of Internal Medicine* 117 (1992): 257.

Fischl, M. A., Uttamchandani, R. B., Daikos, G. L., Poblete, R. B., Moreno, J. N., Reyes, R. R., Boota, A. M., Thompson, L. M., Cleary, T. J., and Lai, S. "An Outbreak of Tuberculosis Caused by Multidrug-Resistant Tubercle Baccilli among Patients with HIV Infection." *Annals of Internal Medicine* 117 (1992): 177.

Jereb, J. A., Kelly, G. D., Dooley, S. W., Jr., Cauthen, G. M., and Snider, D. E., Jr. "Tuberculosis Morbidity in the United States: Final Data, 1990." *Morbidity and Mortality Weekly Report* 40, SS-3 (1992): 23.

Levin, A. C., Gums, J. G., and Grauer, K. "Tuberculosis." *Postgraduate Medicine* 93 (1993): 46.

10 Sexually transmitted diseases

Centers for Disease Control. "Summary of Notifiable Diseases, United States, 1992." *Morbidity and Mortality Weekly Report* 41 (1992): 1.

Centers for Disease Control. "Update: Barrier Protection against HIV Infection and Other Sexually Transmitted Diseases." *Morbidity and Mortality Weekly Report* 42 (1993): 589.

Centers for Disease Control and Prevention. "Sexually Transmitted Diseases Treatment Guidelines—2002." *Morbidity and Mortality Weekly Report* 51, RR-6 (2002): 1–80.

Koutsky, L. A., Steven, C. E., Holmes, K. K., Ashley, R. L., Kiviat, N. B., Critchlow, C. W., and Corey, L. "Underdiagnosis of Genital Herpes by Current Clinical and Viral-Isolation Procedures." *New England Journal of Medicine* 326 (1992): 1533.

Krieger, J. N., Jenny, C., Verdon, M., and Siegel, N. "Clinical Manifestations of Trichomoniasis in Men." *Annals of Internal Medicine* 118 (1993): 844.

Morrison, E. A. "Natural History of Cervical Infection with Human Papillomavirus." *Clinical Infectious Diseases* 18 (1994): 172.

11 Hepatitis

American Academy of Pediatrics Committee on Infectious Diseases. "Universal Hepatitis B Immunization." *Pediatrics* 89 (4, pt. 2) (1992): 795.

Bancroft, W. H. "Hepatitis A Vaccine." *New England Journal of Medicine* 327 (1992): 488.

Dindzans, V. J. "Viral Hepatitis: Preexposure and Postexposure Prophylaxis." *Postgraduate Medicine* 92 (1992): 43.

Dodd, R. Y. "The Risk of Transfusion-Transmitted Infection." *New England Journal of Medicine* 327 (1992): 419.

Donahue, J. G., Munoz, A., Ness, P. M., Brown, D. E., Jr., Yawn, D. H., McAllister, H. A., Jr., Reitz, B. A., and Nelson, K. E. "The Declining Risk of Posttransfusion Hepatitis C. Virus Infection." *New England Journal of Medicine* 327 (1992): 369.

Esteban, J. I., Lopez-Talavera, J. C., Genesca, J., Madoz, P., Viladomiu, L., Muniz, E., Martin-Vega, C., Rosell, M., Allende, H., Vidal, X., Gonzalez, A., Hernandez, J. M., Esteban, R., and Guardia, J. "High Rate of Infectivity and Liver Disease in Blood Donors with Antibodies to Hepatitis C Virus." *Annals of Internal Medicine* 115 (1991): 443.

Gerberding, J. L., and Henderson, D. K. "Management of Occupational Exposures to Bloodborne Pathogens: Hepatitis B Virus, Hepatitis C Virus, and Human Immunodeficiency Virus." *Clinical Infectious Diseases* 14 (1992): 1179.

Lerman, Y., Shohat, T., Ashkenazi, S., Almog, R., Heering, S. L., and Shemer, J. "Efficacy of Different Doses of Immune Serum Globulin in the Prevention of Hepatitis A: A Three-Year Prospective Study." *Clinical Infectious Diseases* 17 (1993): 411.

Melbye, M., Biggar, R. J., Wantzin, P., Krogsgaard, K., Ebbesen, P., and Becker, N. G. "Sexual Transmission of Hepatitis C Virus: Cohort Study (1981–89) among European Homosexual Men." *British Medical Journal* 301 (1990): 210.

12 HIV infection and AIDS

Centers for Disease Control. "Update: Barrier Protection against HIV Infection and Other Sexually Transmitted Diseases." *Morbidity and Mortality Weekly Report* 42 (1993): 589.

Centers for Disease Control. "Recommended Infection-Control Practices for Dentistry, 1993." *Morbidity and Mortality Weekly Report* 42, RR-8 (1993): 1.

Centers for Disease Control. "Human Immunodeficiency Virus Transmission in Household Settings—United States." *Morbidity and Mortality Weekly Report* 43 (1994): 347.

Fitzgibbon, J. E., Gaur, S., Frenkel, L. D., Laraque, F., Edlin, B. R., and Dubin, D. T. "Transmission from One Child to Another of Human Immunodeficiency Virus Type 1 with a Zidovudine-Resistance Mutation." *New England Journal of Medicine* 329 (1993): 1835.

Fahey, B. J., Beekmann, S. E., Schmidt, J. M., Fredio, J. M., and Henderson, D. K. "Managing Occupational Exposures to HIV-1 in the Healthcare Workplace." *Infection Control and Hospital Epidemiology* 14 (1993): 405.

Gershon, R. M., Vlahov, D., and Nelson, K. E. "HIV Infection Risk to Non–Health Care Workers." *American Industrial Hygiene Association Journal* 51 (1990): A807.

Gershon, R. M., Vlahov, D., and Nelson, K. E. "The Risk of Transmission of HIV-1 through Nonpercutaneous Nonsexual Modes: A Review." *AIDS* 4 (1990): 645.

Klein, R. S., and Friedland, G. H. "Transmission of Human Immunodeficieny Virus Type 1 (HIV-1) by Exposure to Blood: Defining the Risk." *Annals of Internal Medicine* 113 (1990): 729.

Kuhn, L., Stein, Z. A., Thomas, P. A., Singh, T., and Tsai, W. "Maternal-Infant HIV Transmission and Circumstances of Delivery." *American Journal of Public Health* 84 (1994): 1110.

Longfield, J. N., Brundage, J., Badger, G., Vire, D., Milazzo, M., Ray, K., Gemmill, R., Magruder, C., Oster, C. N., and Roberts, C. "Look-Back Investigation after Human Immunodeficiency Virus Seroconversion in a Pediatric Dentist." *Journal of Infectious Diseases* 169 (1994): 1.

Rich, J. D., Buck, A., Tuomala, R. E., and Kazanjian, P. H. "Transmission of Human Immunodeficiency Virus Infection Presumed to Have Occurred via Female Homosexual Contact." *Clinical Infectious Diseases* 17 (1993): 1003.

Schaffner, W. "Surgeons with HIV Infection: The Risk to Patients." *Journal of Hospital Infection* 18, Supp. A (1991): 191.

Vincenzi, I. "A Longitudinal Study of Human Immunodeficiency Virus Transmission by Heterosexual Partners." *New England Journal of Medicine* 331 (1994): 341.

Webb, P. A., Happ, C. M., Maupin, G. O., Johnson, B.J.B., Ou, C., and Monath, T. P. "Potential for Insect Transmission of HIV: Experimental Exposure of *Cimex hemipterus* and *Toxorhynchites amboinensis* to Human Immunodeficiency Virus." *Journal of Infectious Diseases* 160 (1989): 970.

13 Special persons and special situations

Bell, D.S.H. "Lower Limb Problems in Diabetic Patients." *Postgraduate Medicine* 89 (1991): 237.

Cole, J. T., and Flaum, M. A. "Post-Splenectomy Infections." *Southern Medical Journal* 85 (1992): 1220.

Dejani, A. S., Bisno, A. L., Chung, K. J., Durack, D. T., Freed, M., Gerber, M. A., Karchmer, A. W., Millard, H. D., Rahimtoola, S., Shulman, S. T., Watanakunakorn, C., and Taubert, K. A. "Prevention of Bacterial Endocarditis: Recommendations by the American Heart Association." *Journal of the American Medical Association* 264 (1990): 2919.

McGowan, J. S., Chesney, P. J., Crossley, K. B., and LaForce, F. M. "Guidelines for the Use of Systemic Glucocorticosteroids in the Management of Selected Infections." *Journal of Infectious Diseases* 165 (1992): 1.

Rimola, A., Bory, F., Teres, J., Perez-Ayuso, R. M., Arroyo, V., and Rodes, J. "Oral, Nonabsorbable Antibiotics Prevent Infection in Cirrhotics with Gastrointestinal Hemorrhage." *Hepatology* 5 (1985): 463.

Rubin, R. H., Wolfson, J. S., Cosimi, A. B., and Tolkoff-Rubin, N. E. "Infection in the Renal Transplant Recipient." *American Journal of Medicine* 70 (1981): 405.

Singh, N., Gayowski, T., Yu, V. L., and Wagener, M. "Trimethoprim-Sulfamethoxazole for the Prevention of Spontaneous Bacterial Peritonitis in Cirrhosis: A Randomized Trial." *Annals of Internal Medicine* 122 (1995): 595.

14 How to avoid infections if you have HIV

Carr, A., Tindall, B., Brew, B. J., Marriott, D. J., Harkness, J. L., Penny, R., and Cooper, D. A. "Low-Dose Trimethoprim-Sulfamethoxazole Prophylaxis for Toxoplasmic Encephalitis in Patients with AIDS." *Annals of Internal Medicine* 117 (1992): 106.

Centers for Disease Control. "Management of Persons Exposed to Multidrug-Resistant Tuberculosis." *Morbidity and Mortality Weekly Report* 41 (1992): 61.

Coronado, V. G., Beck-Sague, C. M., Pearson, M. L., Valway, S. E., Pineda, M. R., and Jarvis, W. R. "Multidrug-Resistant *Mycobacterium tuberculosis* among Patients with HIV Infection." *Infectious Diseases in Clinical Practice* 2 (1993): 297.

Galgiani, J. N. "Coccidioidomycosis." *Infectious Diseases in Clinical Practice* 1 (1992): 357.

Gallant, J. E., Moore, R. D., Richman, D. D., Keruly, J., and Chaisson, R. E. "Incidence and Natural History of Cytomegalovirus Disease in Patients with Advanced Human Immunodeficiency Disease Treated with Zidovudine." *Journal of Infectious Diseases* 166 (1992): 1223.

Girard, P., Landman, R., Gaudebout, C., Olivares, R., Saimot, A. G., Jelazko, P., Gaudebout, C., Certain, A., Boue, F., Bouvet, E., Lecompte, T., and Couland, J. "Dapsone-Pyrimethamine Compared with Aerosolized Pentamidine as Primary Prophylaxis against *Pneumocystis carinii* Pneumonia and Toxoplasmosis in HIV Infections." *New England Journal of Medicine* 328 (1993): 1514.

Grant, I. H., Gold, J.W.M., Rosenblum, M., Niedzwiecki, D., and Armstrong, D. "*Toxoplasma gondii* Serology in HIV-Infected Patients: The Development of Central Nervous System Toxoplasmosis in AIDS." *AIDS* 4 (1990): 519.

Hardy, W. D., Feinberg, J., Finkelstein, D. M., Power, M. E., He, W., Kaczka, C., Frame, P. T., Holmes, M., Waskin, H., Fass, R. J., Powderly, W. G., Steigbigel, R. T., Zuger, A., and Holzman, R. S. "A Controlled Trial of Trimethoprim-Sulfamethoxazole or Aerosolized Pentamidine for Secondary Prophylaxis of *Pneumocystis carinii* Pneumonia in Patients with the Acquired Immunodeficiency Syndrome." *New England Journal of Medicine* 327 (1992): 1842.

Hoover, D. R., Saah, A. J., and Phair, J. "Clinical Manifestations of AIDS in the Era of Pneumocystis Prophylaxis: Multicenter AIDS Cohort Study." *New England Journal of Medicine* 329 (1993): 1922.

Jacobsen, M. A., Besch, C. L., Child, C., Hafner, R., Matts, K. M., Wentworth, D. N., Neaton, J. D., Abrams, D., Rimland, D., Perez, G., Grant, I. H., Saravolatz, L. D., Brown, L. S., and Deyton, L. "Primary Prophylaxis with Pyrimethamine for Toxoplasmic Encephalitis in Patients with Advanced Human Immunodeficiency Virus Disease: Results of a Randomized Trial." *Journal of Infectious Diseases* 169 (1994): 384.

Jewett, J. F., and Hecht, F. M. "Preventive Health Care for Adults with HIV Infection." *Journal of the American Medical Association* 269 (1993): 1144.

Leighty, J. C. "Strategies for Control of Toxoplasmosis." *Journal of the Veterinary Medical Association* 196 (1990): 281.

Markowitz, N., Hansen, N. I., Wilcosky, T. C., Hopewell, P. C., Glassroth, J., Kvale, P. A., Mangura, B. T., Osmond, D., Wallace, J. M., Rosen, M. J., and Reichman, L. B. "Tuberculin and Anergy Testing in HIV-Seropositive and HIV-Seronegative Persons." *Annals of Internal Medicine* 119 (1993): 185.

Moreno, S., Baraia-Extaburu, J., Bouza, E., Parras, F., Pérez-Tascón, M., Miralles, P., Vincent, T., Alberdi, J., Cosín, J., and López-Gay, D. "Risk for Developing Tuberculosis among Anergic Patients Infected with HIV." *Annals of Internal Medicine* 119 (1993): 194.

Newton, J. A., Olson, P., Tasker, S. A., Bone, W. D., Nguyen, M. T., and Oldfield, E. C. "Weekly Fluconazole for the Suppression of Recurrent Thursh in HIV-Seropositive Patients: Impact on the Incidence of Disseminated Cryptococcal Infection." Infectious Disease Society of America Annual Meeting, October 16, 1993, New Orleans, program abstract number 194.

Nightingale, S. D., Byrd, L. T., Southern, P. M., Jockusch, J. D., Cal, S. X., and Wynne, B. A. "Incidence of *Mycobacterium avium-intracellulare* Complex Bacteremia in Human Immunodeficiency Virus–Positive Patients." *Journal of Infectious Diseases* 165 (1992): 1082.

Nightingale, S. D., Cal, S. X., Peterson, D. M., Loss, S. D., Gamble, B.A., Watson, D. A., Manzones, C. P., Baker, J. E., and Jockusch, J. D. "Primary Prophylaxis with Fluconazole against Systemic Fungal Infections in HIV-Positive Patients." *AIDS* 6 (1992): 191.

Nightingale, S. D., Cameron, D. W., Gordin, F. M., Sullam, P. M., Cohn, D. L., Chaisson, R. E., Eron, L. J., Sparti, P. D., Bihari, B., Kaufman, D. L., Stern,

J. J., Pearce, D. D., Weinberg, W. G., LaMarca, A., and Siegal, F. P. "Two Controlled Trials of Rifabutin Prophylaxis against *Mycobacterium avium* Complex Infection in AIDS." *New England Journal of Medicine* 329 (1993): 828.

Pape, J. W., Jean, S. S., Ho, J. L., Hafner, A., and Johnson, W. D., Jr. "Effect of Isoniazid Prophylaxis on Incidence of Active Tuberculosis and Progression of HIV Infection." *The Lancet* 342 (1993): 268.

Phair, J., Munoz, A., Detels, R., Kaslow, R., Rinaldo, C., Saah, A., and the Multicenter AIDS Cohort Study Group. "The Risk of *Pneumocystis carinii* Pneumonia among Men Infected with Human Immunodeficiency Virus Type 1." *New England Journal of Medicine* 322 (1990): 161.

Powderly, W. G. "Cryptococcal Meningitis and AIDS." *Clinical Infectious Diseases* 17 (1993): 837.

Rabkin, C. S., Hatzakis, A., Griffiths, P. D., and Pillay, D. "Cytomegalovirus Infection and Risk of AIDS in Human Immunodeficiency Virus–Infected Hemophilia Patients." *Journal of Infectious Diseases* 168 (1993): 1260.

Raven, P., Lundgren, J. D., Kjaeldgaard, P., Holten-Anderson, W., Hojlyng, N., Nielsen, J. O., and Gaub, J. "Nosocomial Outbreak of Cryptosporidiosis in AIDS Patients." *British Medical Journal* 302 (1991): 277.

Schneider, M.M.E., Hoepelman, A.I.M., Schattenkerk, J.K.M.E., Nielsen, T. L., Graaf, Y., Frissen, J.P.H.J., Ende, I.M.E., Kolsters, A.F.P., and Borleffs, J.C.C. "A Controlled Trial of Aerosolized Pentamidine or Trimethoprim-Sulfamethoxazole as Primary Prophylaxis against *Pneumocystis carinii* Pneumonia in Patients with Human Immunodeficiency Virus Infection." *New England Journal of Medicine* 327 (1992): 1836.

Schooley, R. T. "Cytomegalovirus in the Setting of Infection with Human Immunodeficiency Virus." *Reviews of Infectious Diseases* 12, Supp. 7 (1990): S811.

Smith, P. D., Quinn, T. C. , Strober, W., Janoff, E. N., and Masur, H. "Gastrointestinal Infections in AIDS." *Annals of Internal Medicine* 116 (1992): 63.

Terry, S. "Drinking Water Comes to a Boil." *New York Times Magazine,* September 26, 1993, p. 43ff.

USPHS/IDSA Prevention of Opportunistic Infections Working Group. "1999 USPHS/IDSA Guidelines for the Prevention of Opportunistic Infections in Persons Infected with Human Immunodeficiency Virus." *Clinical Infectious Diseases* 30 (2000): S29–S65.

Wheat, L. J. "Histoplasmosis in AIDS." *AIDS Clinical Care* 4 (1992): l.

15 *If you are pregnant*

Adler, S. P. "Cytomegalovirus and Pregnancy." *Current Opinion in Obstetrics and Gynecology* 4 (1992): 670.

Alford, C. A., Stagno, S., Pass, R. F., and Britt, W. J. "Congenital and Perinatal Cytomegalovirus Infections." *Review of Infectious Diseases* 12, Supp. 7 (1990): S745.

Bakht, F. R., and Gentry, L. O. "Toxoplasmosis in Pregnancy: An Emerging Concern for Family Physicians." *American Family Physician* 45 (1992): 1683.

Brunell, P. A. "Varicella in Pregnancy, the Fetus, and the Newborn: Problems in Management." *Journal of Infectious Diseases* 166, Supp. 1 (1992): S42.

Centers for Disease Control. "1993 Sexually Transmitted Diseases Treatment Guidelines." *Morbidity and Mortality Weekly Report* 42, RR-14 (1993): 37.

Centers for Disease Control. "Update: Foodborne Listeriosis—United States, 1988–1990." *Morbidity and Mortality Weekly Report* 41 (1992): 251.

Daffos, F., Forestier, F., Capella-Pavlovsky, M., Thulliez, P., Aufrant, C., Valenti, D., and Cox, W. L. "Prenatal Management of 746 Pregnancies at Risk for Congenital Toxoplasmosis." *New England Journal of Medicine* 318 (1988): 271.

Dobbins, J. G., Stewart, J. A., and Demmier, G. J. "Surveillance of Congenital Cytomegalovirus Disease, 1990–1991," in "CDC Surveillance Summaries, April 24, 1992." *Morbidity and Mortality Weekly Report* 41 (1992): 35.

Gellin, B. G., and Broome, C. V. "Listeriosis." *Journal of the American Medical Association* 261 (1989): 1313.

Greenspoon, J. S., Wilcox, J. G., and Kirschbaum, T. H. "Group B Streptococcus: The Effectiveness of Screening and Chemoprophylaxis." *Obstetrical and Gynecological Survey* 46 (1991): 499.

Gordon, M. C., and Hankins, G.D.V. "Urinary Tract Infections and Pregnancy." *Comprehensive Therapy* 15 (1989): 52.

Jeannel, D., Costagliola, D., Niel, G., Hubert, B., and Danis, M. "What Is Known about the Prevention of Congenital Toxoplasmosis?" *Lancet* 336 (1990): 359.

Lynch, L., and Ghidini, A. "Perinatal Infections." *Current Opinions in Obstetrics and Gynecology* 5 (1993): 24.

Mateo, J. R., and Sever, J. L. "Perinatally Acquired Infections and Screening." *Current Opinions in Obstetrics and Gynecology* 2 (1990): 662.

Miller, E. "Rubella Infection in Pregnancy: Remaining Problems." *British Journal of Obstetrics and Gynaecology* 96 (1989): 887.

Pastuszak, A. L., Levy, M., Schick, B., Zuber, C., Feldkamp, M., Gladstone, J., Bar-Levy, F., Jackson, E., Donnenfeld, A., Meschino, W., and Koren, G. "Outcome after Maternal Varicella Infection in the First 20 Weeks of Pregnancy." *New England Journal of Medicine* 330 (1994): 901.

Prober, C. G., Corey, L., Brown, Z. A., Hensleigh, P. A., Frenkel, L. M., Bryson, Y. J., Whitley, R. J., and Arvin, A. M. "The Management of Pregnancies Complicated by Genital Infections with Herpes Simplex Virus." *Clinical Infectious Diseases* 15 (1992): 1031–1038.

Remington, J. S., and Klein, J. O., eds. *Infectious Diseases of the Fetus and Newborn Infant.* 3rd ed. Philadelphia: W. B. Saunders, 1990.

Schuchat, A., Swaminathan, B., and Broome, C. "Epidemiology of Human Listeriosis." *Clinical Microbiology Review* 4 (1991): 169.

Sinnott, J. T., and Cacciatore, M. L. "Measles in Pregnancy: Physician on the Spot." *Infections in Medicine,* August 1992, p. 45.

Skogberg, K., Syjanen, J., Jahkola, M., Renkonen, O., Paavonen, J., Ahonen, J., Kontiainen, S., Ruutu, P., and Valtonen, V. "Clinical Presentation and Outcome of Listeriosis in Patients with and without Immunosuppressive Therapy." *Clinical Infectious Diseases* 14 (1992): 815.

16 In the hospital

Centers for Disease Control. "Public Focus: Surveillance, Prevention and Control of Nosocomial Infections." *Morbidity and Mortality Weekly Report* 41 (1992): 783.

Dodd, R. Y. "The Risk of Transfusion-Transmitted Infection." *New England Journal of Medicine* 237 (1992): 419.

Doebbeling, B. N., Stanley, G. L., Sheetz, C. T., Pfaller, M. A., Houston, A. K., Ning Li, L. A., and Wenzel, R. P. "Comparative Efficacy of Alternative Hand-Washing Agents in Reducing Nosocomial Infections in Intensive Care Units." *New England Journal of Medicine* 327 (1992): 88.

Goldman, D. "Hand-Washing and Nosocomial Infections." *New England Journal of Medicine* 327 (1992): 120.

Kluytmans, J.A.J.W., Mouton, J. W., Ijzerman, E.P.F., Vandenbroucke-Grauls, C.M.J.E., Maat, A.W.P.M., Wagenvoort, J.H.T., and Verbrugh, H. A. "Nasal Carriage of *Staphylococcus aureus* as a Major Risk Factor for Wound Infections after Cardiac Surgery." *Journal of Infectious Diseases* 171 (1995): 216.

17 Emerging infections

Centers for Disease Control and Prevention. "Outbreak of West Nile-like Viral Encephalitis—New York, 1999." *Morbidity and Mortality Weekly Report* 48 (1999): 845–849.

Centers for Disease Control and Prevention. "Probable variant Creutzfeldt-Jakob disease in a U.S. resident—Florida, 2002." *Morbidity and Mortality Weekly Report* 51 (2002): 927–929.

Centers for Disease Control and Prevention. "Fatal Degenerative Neurologic Illnesses in Men Who Participated in Wild Game Feasts—Wisconsin, 2002." *Morbidity and Mortality Weekly Report* 52 (2003): 125–127.

Fradin, M. S., and Day, J. F. "Comparative Efficacy of Insect Repellents against Mosquito Bites." *New England Journal of Medicine* 347 (2002): 13–18.

Goddard, L. B., Roth, A. E., Reisen, W. K., and Scott, T. W. "Vector Competence of California Mosquitoes for West Nile virus." *Emerging Infectious Diseases* 12 (2002): 1385–1388.

Loeb, M., McGeer, A., Henry, B., Ofner, M., Rose, D., Hlywka, T., Levie, J., McQueen, J., Smith, S., Moss, L., Smith, A., Green, K., and Walter, S. D. "SARS among Critical Care Nurses, Toronto." *Emerging Infectious Diseases* 10 (2004): 251–5.

Murphy, M. E., Montemarano, A. D., Debboun, M., and Gupta, R. "The Effect of Sunscreen on the Efficacy of Insect Repellent: A Clinical Trial." *Journal of the American Academy of Dermatology* 43 (2000): 219–22.

Nash, D., Mostashari, F., Fine, A., Miller, J., O'Leary, D., Murray, K., Huang, A., Rosenberg, A., Greenberg, A., Sherman, M., Wong, S., Campbell, G. L., Roehrig, J. T., Gubler, D. J., Shieh, W., Zaki, S., Smith, P., and Layton, M. "The Outbreak of West Nile Virus Infection in the New York City Area in 1999." *New England Journal of Medicine* 344 (2001): 1807–1814.

Will, R. G., Ironside, J. W., Zeidler, M., Cousens, S. N., Estibeiro, K., Alperovitch, A., Poser, S., Pocchiari, M., Hofman, A., and Smith, P. G. "A New Variant of Creutzfeldt-Jakob Disease in the UK." *Lancet* 347 (1996): 921–5.

Wu, J., Xu, F., Zhou, W., Feikin, D. R., Lin, C., He, X., Zhu, Z., Liang, W., Chin, D. P., and Schuchat, A. "Risk Factors for SARS among Persons without Known Contact with SARS Patients: Beijing, China." *Emerging Infectious Diseases* 10 (2004): 210–216.

18 Bioterrorism

Henderson, D. A., Inglesby, T. V., Bartlett, J. G., Ascher, M. S., Eitzen, E., Jahrling, P. B., Hauer J., Layton, M., McDade, J., Osterholm, M. T., O'Toole, T., Parker, G., Pen, T., Russell, P. K., and Tonat, K., for the Working Group on Civilian Biodefense. "Smallpox as a Biological Weapon: Medical and Public Health Management." *Journal of the American Medical Association* 281 (1999): 2127–2137.

Inglesby, T. V., Dennis, D. T., Henderson, D. A., Bartlett, J. G., Ascher, M. S., Eitzen, B., Fine, A. D., Friedlander, A. M., Hauer, J., Koerner, J. F., Layton, M., McDade, J., Osterholm, M. R., O'Toole, T., Parker, G., Perl, T. M., Russell, P. K., Schoch-Spana, M., and Tonat, K. "Plague as a Biological Weapon." *Journal of the American Medical Association* 238 (2000): 2281–2290.

Jernigan, J. A., Stephens, D. S., Ashford, D. A., Omenaca, C., Topiel, M. S., Galbraith, M., Tapper, M., Fisk, T. L., Zaki, S., Popovic, T., Meyer, R. F., Quinn, C. P., Harper, S. A., Fridkin, S. K., Sejvar, J. J., Shepard, C. W., McConnell, M., Guarner, J., Shieh, W., Maleki, J. M. Gerberding J. L., Hughes, J. M., and Perkins, B. A., "Bioterrorism-related Inhalational Anthrax: The first 10 Cases Reported in the United States." *Emerging Infectious Diseases* 6 (2001): 933–944.

Index

absolute neutrophil count (ANC), 189–191
Access America Service Corporation, 103
achlorhydria, 103
acquired immune deficiency syndrome, *see* AIDS
acyclovir (Zovirax), 39, 148, 214–215, 242
Africa, 84, 89, 92, 96, 100, 132–133, 161, 163, 211
African sleeping sickness, 87
AIDS: and bacterial pneumonia, 204; and candidiasis, 205–207, 224; and CD4 count, 203–204; and CMV, 205, 207–209, 211, 224; and coccidioidomycosis, 209; and cryptococcosis, 210, 224; and *Cryptosporidium*, 74, 213; and diarrhea, 61, 210–213; and diet, 223, 225; and exercise, 223, 225; and helper cell count, 203–204; and hepatitis B, 213–214; and hepatitis C, 214; and herpes simplex virus, 214–215; and histoplasmosis, 215–216; and MAC (*Mycobacterium avium* complex), 202, 204, 211, 217, 224; and opportunistic infections (OIs), 202–204; and *Pneumocystis carinii* pneumonia (PCP), 202, 204, 217–219; and *Salmonella*, 212–213; and sex, 209, 223, 225; and shingles, 215; and smoking, 223; and syphilis, 219; and toxoplasmosis, 202, 204, 219–221; and tuberculosis (TB), 138, 221–223. *See also* HIV infection
alcohol, 109, 137, 143, 172
amantadine (Symmetrel), 114–115
amebic dysentery, 5–6, 80, 106
amoxicillin, 145, 285

ampicillin, 237, 285
ANC (absolute neutrophil count), 189–191
animal bites, 34–36, 286
anisakiasis, 68
antacid medicines, 59, 211, 245
anthrax, 270–273, 275
Aralen, *see* chloroquine
Argentina, 85
Arizona, 5, 56, 116, 118, 209
Arkansas, 56
ascorbic acid, *see* vitamin C
aspergillosis, 190, 193, 195
athlete's foot, 36–37
Australia, 56, 79, 158
azithromycin (Zithromax), 144–145
AZT (Retrovir, zidovudine), 172–174, 204

babesiosis, 56, 196
Bacille Calmette-Guérin, *see* BCG
Bacillus cereus, 62–63
Bactrim, *see* trimethoprim/sulfamethoxazole
Bactroban, *see* mupirocin
Bangladesh, 58
bats, 98, 216, 286
BCG (Bacille Calmette-Guérin), 132–133, 278
beef, 57, 61–64
Bell's palsy, 46
Betadine, *see* povidone-iodine
bioterrorism, 270–275
BioWatch, 272
birds, 76, 118, 210, 216
bites, 34–36, 97, 197, 225
bleach, 76, 169–170, 172, 177
blood transfusions, 170–171, 252–253
boils, 33–34, 67, 73, 187, 198, 247
Borrelia burgdorferi, 25–49, 55
Boston, Mass., 238
botulism, 58, 62–63, 66, 69, 271, 275

About the author

Winkler G. Weinberg, M.D., is Chief of Infectious Diseases for the Southeast Permanente Medical Group (a section of the health maintenance organization Kaiser Permanente) and is actively engaged in research on infectious diseases. Dr. Weinberg received his M.D. degree from the Medical College of Georgia and completed a residency in internal medicine at Georgetown University. During his service as lieutenant commander in the U.S. Navy Medical Corps, he completed a fellowship in infectious diseases at the Uniformed Services University of the Health Services and coordinated the sexually transmitted disease program at the the Navy's regional medical center at Subic Bay. He is a Diplomate in the Specialty of Infectious Disease and a Diplomate of the American Board of Internal Medicine. He lives with his wife in Atlanta, Georgia, and they have two grown children. This book grows out of his stewardship of a busy travel medicine clinic and his daily experience caring for patients with infectious diseases.